AF 778600

Family Practice Exam

SECRETS

Study Guide

Your Key to Exam Success

FP Test Review for the
Family Practice Board Exam

Dear Future Exam Success Story:

First of all, **THANK YOU** for purchasing Mometrix study materials!

Second, congratulations! You are one of the few determined test-takers who are committed to doing whatever it takes to excel on your exam. **You have come to the right place.** We developed these study materials with one goal in mind: to deliver you the information you need in a format that's concise and easy to use.

In addition to optimizing your guide for the content of the test, we've outlined our recommended steps for breaking down the preparation process into small, attainable goals so you can make sure you stay on track.

We've also analyzed the entire test-taking process, identifying the most common pitfalls and showing how you can overcome them and be ready for any curveball the test throws you.

Standardized testing is one of the biggest obstacles on your road to success, which only increases the importance of doing well in the high-pressure, high-stakes environment of test day. Your results on this test could have a significant impact on your future, and this guide provides the information and practical advice to help you achieve your full potential on test day.

Your success is our success

We would love to hear from you! If you would like to share the story of your exam success or if you have any questions or comments in regard to our products, please contact us at **800-673-8175** or **support@mometrix.com**.

Thanks again for your business and we wish you continued success!

Sincerely,
The Mometrix Test Preparation Team

Need more help? Check out our flashcards at:
http://MometrixFlashcards.com/FamilyPractice

Written and edited by the Mometrix Exam Secrets Test Prep Team
Printed in the United States of America

TABLE OF CONTENTS

Introduction

Thank you for purchasing this resource! You have made the choice to prepare yourself for a test that could have a huge impact on your future, and this guide is designed to help you be fully ready for test day. Obviously, it's important to have a solid understanding of the test material, but you also need to be prepared for the unique environment and stressors of the test, so that you can perform to the best of your abilities.

For this purpose, the first section that appears in this guide is the **Secret Keys**. We've devoted countless hours to meticulously researching what works and what doesn't, and we've boiled down our findings to the five most impactful steps you can take to improve your performance on the test. We start at the beginning with study planning and move through the preparation process, all the way to the testing strategies that will help you get the most out of what you know when you're finally sitting in front of the test.

We recommend that you start preparing for your test as far in advance as possible. However, if you've bought this guide as a last-minute study resource and only have a few days before your test, we recommend that you skip over the first two Secret Keys since they address a long-term study plan.

If you struggle with **test anxiety**, we strongly encourage you to check out our recommendations for how you can overcome it. Test anxiety is a formidable foe, but it can be beaten, and we want to make sure you have the tools you need to defeat it.

Secret Key #1 – Plan Big, Study Small

There's a lot riding on your performance. If you want to ace this test, you're going to need to keep your skills sharp and the material fresh in your mind. You need a plan that lets you review everything you need to know while still fitting in your schedule. We'll break this strategy down into three categories.

Information Organization

Start with the information you already have: the official test outline. From this, you can make a complete list of all the concepts you need to cover before the test. Organize these concepts into groups that can be studied together, and create a list of any related vocabulary you need to learn so you can brush up on any difficult terms. You'll want to keep this vocabulary list handy once you actually start studying since you may need to add to it along the way.

Time Management

Once you have your set of study concepts, decide how to spread them out over the time you have left before the test. Break your study plan into small, clear goals so you have a manageable task for each day and know exactly what you're doing. Then just focus on one small step at a time. When you manage your time this way, you don't need to spend hours at a time studying. Studying a small block of content for a short period each day helps you retain information better and avoid stressing over how much you have left to do. You can relax knowing that you have a plan to cover everything in time. In order for this strategy to be effective though, you have to start studying early and stick to your schedule. Avoid the exhaustion and futility that comes from last-minute cramming!

Study Environment

The environment you study in has a big impact on your learning. Studying in a coffee shop, while probably more enjoyable, is not likely to be as fruitful as studying in a quiet room. It's important to keep distractions to a minimum. You're only planning to study for a short block of time, so make the most of it. Don't pause to check your phone or get up to find a snack. It's also important to **avoid multitasking**. Research has consistently shown that multitasking will make your studying dramatically less effective. Your study area should also be comfortable and well-lit so you don't have the distraction of straining your eyes or sitting on an uncomfortable chair.

The time of day you study is also important. You want to be rested and alert. Don't wait until just before bedtime. Study when you'll be most likely to comprehend and remember. Even better, if you know what time of day your test will be, set that time aside for study. That way your brain will be used to working on that subject at that specific time and you'll have a better chance of recalling information.

Finally, it can be helpful to team up with others who are studying for the same test. Your actual studying should be done in as isolated an environment as possible, but the work of organizing the information and setting up the study plan can be divided up. In between study sessions, you can discuss with your teammates the concepts that you're all studying and quiz each other on the details. Just be sure that your teammates are as serious about the test as you are. If you find that your study time is being replaced with social time, you might need to find a new team.

Secret Key #2 – Make Your Studying Count

You're devoting a lot of time and effort to preparing for this test, so you want to be absolutely certain it will pay off. This means doing more than just reading the content and hoping you can remember it on test day. It's important to make every minute of study count. There are two main areas you can focus on to make your studying count:

Retention

It doesn't matter how much time you study if you can't remember the material. You need to make sure you are retaining the concepts. To check your retention of the information you're learning, try recalling it at later times with minimal prompting. Try carrying around flashcards and glance at one or two from time to time or ask a friend who's also studying for the test to quiz you.

To enhance your retention, look for ways to put the information into practice so that you can apply it rather than simply recalling it. If you're using the information in practical ways, it will be much easier to remember. Similarly, it helps to solidify a concept in your mind if you're not only reading it to yourself but also explaining it to someone else. Ask a friend to let you teach them about a concept you're a little shaky on (or speak aloud to an imaginary audience if necessary). As you try to summarize, define, give examples, and answer your friend's questions, you'll understand the concepts better and they will stay with you longer. Finally, step back for a big picture view and ask yourself how each piece of information fits with the whole subject. When you link the different concepts together and see them working together as a whole, it's easier to remember the individual components.

Finally, practice showing your work on any multi-step problems, even if you're just studying. Writing out each step you take to solve a problem will help solidify the process in your mind, and you'll be more likely to remember it during the test.

Modality

Modality simply refers to the means or method by which you study. Choosing a study modality that fits your own individual learning style is crucial. No two people learn best in exactly the same way, so it's important to know your strengths and use them to your advantage.

For example, if you learn best by visualization, focus on visualizing a concept in your mind and draw an image or a diagram. Try color-coding your notes, illustrating them, or creating symbols that will trigger your mind to recall a learned concept. If you learn best by hearing or discussing information, find a study partner who learns the same way or read aloud to yourself. Think about how to put the information in your own words. Imagine that you are giving a lecture on the topic and record yourself so you can listen to it later.

For any learning style, flashcards can be helpful. Organize the information so you can take advantage of spare moments to review. Underline key words or phrases. Use different colors for different categories. Mnemonic devices (such as creating a short list in which every item starts with the same letter) can also help with retention. Find what works best for you and use it to store the information in your mind most effectively and easily.

Secret Key #3 – Practice the Right Way

Your success on test day depends not only on how many hours you put into preparing, but also on whether you prepared the right way. It's good to check along the way to see if your studying is paying off. One of the most effective ways to do this is by taking practice tests to evaluate your progress. Practice tests are useful because they show exactly where you need to improve. Every time you take a practice test, pay special attention to these three groups of questions:

- The questions you got wrong
- The questions you had to guess on, even if you guessed right
- The questions you found difficult or slow to work through

This will show you exactly what your weak areas are, and where you need to devote more study time. Ask yourself why each of these questions gave you trouble. Was it because you didn't understand the material? Was it because you didn't remember the vocabulary? Do you need more repetitions on this type of question to build speed and confidence? Dig into those questions and figure out how you can strengthen your weak areas as you go back to review the material.

Additionally, many practice tests have a section explaining the answer choices. It can be tempting to read the explanation and think that you now have a good understanding of the concept. However, an explanation likely only covers part of the question's broader context. Even if the explanation makes sense, **go back and investigate** every concept related to the question until you're positive you have a thorough understanding.

As you go along, keep in mind that the practice test is just that: practice. Memorizing these questions and answers will not be very helpful on the actual test because it is unlikely to have any of the same exact questions. If you only know the right answers to the sample questions, you won't be prepared for the real thing. **Study the concepts** until you understand them fully, and then you'll be able to answer any question that shows up on the test.

It's important to wait on the practice tests until you're ready. If you take a test on your first day of study, you may be overwhelmed by the amount of material covered and how much you need to learn. Work up to it gradually.

On test day, you'll need to be prepared for answering questions, managing your time, and using the test-taking strategies you've learned. It's a lot to balance, like a mental marathon that will have a big impact on your future. Like training for a marathon, you'll need to start slowly and work your way up. When test day arrives, you'll be ready.

Start with the strategies you've read in the first two Secret Keys—plan your course and study in the way that works best for you. If you have time, consider using multiple study resources to get different approaches to the same concepts. It can be helpful to see difficult concepts from more than one angle. Then find a good source for practice tests. Many times, the test website will suggest potential study resources or provide sample tests.

Practice Test Strategy

When you're ready to start taking practice tests, follow this strategy:

1. Take the first test with no time constraints and with your notes and study guide handy. Take your time and focus on applying the strategies you've learned.
2. Take the second practice test open-book as well, but set a timer and practice pacing yourself to finish in time.
3. Take any other practice tests as if it were test day. Set a timer and put away your study materials. Sit at a table or desk in a quiet room, imagine yourself at the testing center, and answer questions as quickly and accurately as possible.
4. Keep repeating step 3 on a regular basis until you run out of practice tests or it's time for the actual test. Your mind will be ready for the schedule and stress of test day, and you'll be able to focus on recalling the material you've learned.

Secret Key #4 – Pace Yourself

Once you're fully prepared for the material on the test, your biggest challenge on test day will be managing your time. Just knowing that the clock is ticking can make you panic even if you have plenty of time left. Work on pacing yourself so you can build confidence against the time constraints of the exam. Pacing is a difficult skill to master, especially in a high-pressure environment, so **practice is vital**.

Set time expectations for your pace based on how much time is available. For example, if a section has 60 questions and the time limit is 30 minutes, you know you have to average 30 seconds or less per question in order to answer them all. Although 30 seconds is the hard limit, set 25 seconds per question as your goal, so you reserve extra time to spend on harder questions. When you budget extra time for the harder questions, you no longer have any reason to stress when those questions take longer to answer.

Don't let this time expectation distract you from working through the test at a calm, steady pace, but keep it in mind so you don't spend too much time on any one question. Recognize that taking extra time on one question you don't understand may keep you from answering two that you do understand later in the test. If your time limit for a question is up and you're still not sure of the answer, mark it and move on, and come back to it later if the time and the test format allow. If the testing format doesn't allow you to return to earlier questions, just make an educated guess; then put it out of your mind and move on.

On the easier questions, be careful not to rush. It may seem wise to hurry through them so you have more time for the challenging ones, but it's not worth missing one if you know the concept and just didn't take the time to read the question fully. Work efficiently but make sure you understand the question and have looked at all of the answer choices, since more than one may seem right at first.

Even if you're paying attention to the time, you may find yourself a little behind at some point. You should speed up to get back on track, but do so wisely. Don't panic; just take a few seconds less on each question until you're caught up. Don't guess without thinking, but do look through the answer choices and eliminate any you know are wrong. If you can get down to two choices, it is often worthwhile to guess from those. Once you've chosen an answer, move on and don't dwell on any that you skipped or had to hurry through. If a question was taking too long, chances are it was one of the harder ones, so you weren't as likely to get it right anyway.

On the other hand, if you find yourself getting ahead of schedule, it may be beneficial to slow down a little. The more quickly you work, the more likely you are to make a careless mistake that will affect your score. You've budgeted time for each question, so don't be afraid to spend that time. Practice an efficient but careful pace to get the most out of the time you have.

Secret Key #5 – Have a Plan for Guessing

When you're taking the test, you may find yourself stuck on a question. Some of the answer choices seem better than others, but you don't see the one answer choice that is obviously correct. What do you do?

The scenario described above is very common, yet most test takers have not effectively prepared for it. Developing and practicing a plan for guessing may be one of the single most effective uses of your time as you get ready for the exam.

In developing your plan for guessing, there are three questions to address:

- When should you start the guessing process?
- How should you narrow down the choices?
- Which answer should you choose?

When to Start the Guessing Process

Unless your plan for guessing is to select C every time (which, despite its merits, is not what we recommend), you need to leave yourself enough time to apply your answer elimination strategies. Since you have a limited amount of time for each question, that means that if you're going to give yourself the best shot at guessing correctly, you have to decide quickly whether or not you will guess.

Of course, the best-case scenario is that you don't have to guess at all, so first, see if you can answer the question based on your knowledge of the subject and basic reasoning skills. Focus on the key words in the question and try to jog your memory of related topics. Give yourself a chance to bring the knowledge to mind, but once you realize that you don't have (or you can't access) the knowledge you need to answer the question, it's time to start the guessing process.

It's almost always better to start the guessing process too early than too late. It only takes a few seconds to remember something and answer the question from knowledge. Carefully eliminating wrong answer choices takes longer. Plus, going through the process of eliminating answer choices can actually help jog your memory.

Summary: Start the guessing process as soon as you decide that you can't answer the question based on your knowledge.

How to Narrow Down the Choices

The next chapter in this book (**Test-Taking Strategies**) includes a wide range of strategies for how to approach questions and how to look for answer choices to eliminate. You will definitely want to read those carefully, practice them, and figure out which ones work best for you. Here though, we're going to address a mindset rather than a particular strategy.

Your chances of guessing an answer correctly depend on how many options you are choosing from.

How many choices you have	How likely you are to guess correctly
5	20%
4	25%
3	33%
2	50%
1	100%

You can see from this chart just how valuable it is to be able to eliminate incorrect answers and make an educated guess, but there are two things that many test takers do that cause them to miss out on the benefits of guessing:

- Accidentally eliminating the correct answer
- Selecting an answer based on an impression

We'll look at the first one here, and the second one in the next section.

To avoid accidentally eliminating the correct answer, we recommend a thought exercise called **the $5 challenge**. In this challenge, you only eliminate an answer choice from contention if you are willing to bet $5 on it being wrong. Why $5? Five dollars is a small but not insignificant amount of money. It's an amount you could afford to lose but wouldn't want to throw away. And while losing $5 once might not hurt too much, doing it twenty times will set you back $100. In the same way, each small decision you make—eliminating a choice here, guessing on a question there—won't by itself impact your score very much, but when you put them all together, they can make a big difference. By holding each answer choice elimination decision to a higher standard, you can reduce the risk of accidentally eliminating the correct answer.

The $5 challenge can also be applied in a positive sense: If you are willing to bet $5 that an answer choice *is* correct, go ahead and mark it as correct.

Summary: Only eliminate an answer choice if you are willing to bet $5 that it is wrong.

Which Answer to Choose

You're taking the test. You've run into a hard question and decided you'll have to guess. You've eliminated all the answer choices you're willing to bet $5 on. Now you have to pick an answer. Why do we even need to talk about this? Why can't you just pick whichever one you feel like when the time comes?

The answer to these questions is that if you don't come into the test with a plan, you'll rely on your impression to select an answer choice, and if you do that, you risk falling into a trap. The test writers know that everyone who takes their test will be guessing on some of the questions, so they intentionally write wrong answer choices to seem plausible. You still have to pick an answer though, and if the wrong answer choices are designed to look right, how can you ever be sure that you're not falling for their trap? The best solution we've found to this dilemma is to take the decision out of your hands entirely. Here is the process we recommend:

Once you've eliminated any choices that you are confident (willing to bet $5) are wrong, select the first remaining choice as your answer.

Whether you choose to select the first remaining choice, the second, or the last, the important thing is that you use some preselected standard. Using this approach guarantees that you will not be enticed into selecting an answer choice that looks right, because you are not basing your decision on how the answer choices look.

This is not meant to make you question your knowledge. Instead, it is to help you recognize the difference between your knowledge and your impressions. There's a huge difference between thinking an answer is right because of what you know, and thinking an answer is right because it looks or sounds like it should be right.

Summary: To ensure that your selection is appropriately random, make a predetermined selection from among all answer choices you have not eliminated.

Test-Taking Strategies

This section contains a list of test-taking strategies that you may find helpful as you work through the test. By taking what you know and applying logical thought, you can maximize your chances of answering any question correctly!

It is very important to realize that every question is different and every person is different: no single strategy will work on every question, and no single strategy will work for every person. That's why we've included all of them here, so you can try them out and determine which ones work best for different types of questions and which ones work best for you.

Question Strategies

Read Carefully

Read the question and answer choices carefully. Don't miss the question because you misread the terms. You have plenty of time to read each question thoroughly and make sure you understand what is being asked. Yet a happy medium must be attained, so don't waste too much time. You must read carefully, but efficiently.

Contextual Clues

Look for contextual clues. If the question includes a word you are not familiar with, look at the immediate context for some indication of what the word might mean. Contextual clues can often give you all the information you need to decipher the meaning of an unfamiliar word. Even if you can't determine the meaning, you may be able to narrow down the possibilities enough to make a solid guess at the answer to the question.

Prefixes

If you're having trouble with a word in the question or answer choices, try dissecting it. Take advantage of every clue that the word might include. Prefixes and suffixes can be a huge help. Usually they allow you to determine a basic meaning. Pre- means before, post- means after, pro - is positive, de- is negative. From prefixes and suffixes, you can get an idea of the general meaning of the word and try to put it into context.

Hedge Words

Watch out for critical hedge words, such as *likely*, *may*, *can*, *sometimes*, *often*, *almost*, *mostly*, *usually*, *generally*, *rarely*, and *sometimes*. Question writers insert these hedge phrases to cover every possibility. Often an answer choice will be wrong simply because it leaves no room for exception. Be on guard for answer choices that have definitive words such as *exactly* and *always*.

Switchback Words

Stay alert for *switchbacks*. These are the words and phrases frequently used to alert you to shifts in thought. The most common switchback words are *but*, *although*, and *however*. Others include *nevertheless, on the other hand, even though, while, in spite of, despite, regardless of.* Switchback words are important to catch because they can change the direction of the question or an answer choice.

Face Value

When in doubt, use common sense. Accept the situation in the problem at face value. Don't read too much into it. These problems will not require you to make wild assumptions. If you have to go beyond creativity and warp time or space in order to have an answer choice fit the question, then you should move on and consider the other answer choices. These are normal problems rooted in reality. The applicable relationship or explanation may not be readily apparent, but it is there for you to figure out. Use your common sense to interpret anything that isn't clear.

Answer Choice Strategies

Answer Selection

The most thorough way to pick an answer choice is to identify and eliminate wrong answers until only one is left, then confirm it is the correct answer. Sometimes an answer choice may immediately seem right, but be careful. The test writers will usually put more than one reasonable answer choice on each question, so take a second to read all of them and make sure that the other choices are not equally obvious. As long as you have time left, it is better to read every answer choice than to pick the first one that looks right without checking the others.

Eliminate Answers

Eliminate answer choices as soon as you realize they are wrong, but make sure you consider all possibilities. If you are eliminating answer choices and realize that the last one you are left with is also wrong, don't panic. Start over and consider each choice again. There may be something you missed the first time that you will realize on the second pass.

Avoid Fact Traps

Don't be distracted by an answer choice that is factually true but doesn't answer the question. You are looking for the choice that answers the question. Stay focused on what the question is asking for so you don't accidentally pick an answer that is true but incorrect. Always go back to the question and make sure the answer choice you've selected actually answers the question and is not merely a true statement.

Extreme Statements

In general, you should avoid answers that put forth extreme actions as standard practice or proclaim controversial ideas as established fact. An answer choice that states the "process should be used in certain situations, if..." is much more likely to be correct than one that states the "process should be discontinued completely." The first is a calm rational statement and doesn't even make a definitive, uncompromising stance, using a hedge word *if* to provide wiggle room, whereas the second choice is a radical idea and far more extreme.

Benchmark

As you read through the answer choices and you come across one that seems to answer the question well, mentally select that answer choice. This is not your final answer, but it's the one that will help you evaluate the other answer choices. The one that you selected is your benchmark or standard for judging each of the other answer choices. Every other answer choice must be compared to your benchmark. That choice is correct until proven otherwise by another answer choice beating it. If you find a better answer, then that one becomes your new benchmark. Once you've decided that no other choice answers the question as well as your benchmark, you have your final answer.

Predict the Answer

Before you even start looking at the answer choices, it is often best to try to predict the answer. When you come up with the answer on your own, it is easier to avoid distractions and traps because you will know exactly what to look for. The right answer choice is unlikely to be word-for-word what you came up with, but it should be a close match. Even if you are confident that you have the right answer, you should still take the time to read each option before moving on.

General Strategies

Tough Questions

If you are stumped on a problem or it appears too hard or too difficult, don't waste time. Move on! Remember though, if you can quickly check for obviously incorrect answer choices, your chances of guessing correctly are greatly improved. Before you completely give up, at least try to knock out a couple of possible answers. Eliminate what you can and then guess at the remaining answer choices before moving on.

Check Your Work

Since you will probably not know every term listed and the answer to every question, it is important that you get credit for the ones that you do know. Don't miss any questions through careless mistakes. If at all possible, try to take a second to look back over your answer selection and make sure you've selected the correct answer choice and haven't made a costly careless mistake (such as marking an answer choice that you didn't mean to mark). This quick double check should more than pay for itself in caught mistakes for the time it costs.

Pace Yourself

It's easy to be overwhelmed when you're looking at a page full of questions; your mind is confused and full of random thoughts, and the clock is ticking down faster than you would like. Calm down and maintain the pace that you have set for yourself. Especially as you get down to the last few minutes of the test, don't let the small numbers on the clock make you panic. As long as you are on track by monitoring your pace, you are guaranteed to have time for each question.

Don't Rush

It is very easy to make errors when you are in a hurry. Maintaining a fast pace in answering questions is pointless if it makes you miss questions that you would have gotten right otherwise. Test writers like to include distracting information and wrong answers that seem right. Taking a little extra time to avoid careless mistakes can make all the difference in your test score. Find a pace that allows you to be confident in the answers that you select.

Keep Moving

Panicking will not help you pass the test, so do your best to stay calm and keep moving. Taking deep breaths and going through the answer elimination steps you practiced can help to break through a stress barrier and keep your pace.

Final Notes

The combination of a solid foundation of content knowledge and the confidence that comes from practicing your plan for applying that knowledge is the key to maximizing your performance on test day. As your foundation of content knowledge is built up and strengthened, you'll find that the strategies included in this chapter become more and more effective in helping you quickly sift through the distractions and traps of the test to isolate the correct answer.

Now it's time to move on to the test content chapters of this book, but be sure to keep your goal in mind. As you read, think about how you will be able to apply this information on the test. If you've already seen sample questions for the test and you have an idea of the question format and style, try to come up with questions of your own that you can answer based on what you're reading. This will give you valuable practice applying your knowledge in the same ways you can expect to on test day.

Good luck and good studying!

Important Preliminary Information

1. Most of the questions will focus on application of your knowledge of Neurology, Cardiology, Physiology, Pathology, Immunology, Microbiology, Dermatology, Pediatrics, Obstetrics/Gynecology, and Musculoskeletal conditions.
2. Use the review guides listed at the following link: https://www.theabfm.org/
3. Contact Information:

   American Board of Family Medicine, Inc.
   2228 Young Drive, Lexington, Kentucky 40505-4294
   Phone 859-269-5626/888-995-5700
   Email help@theabfm.org

Allergy and Immunology

Eczema

Eczema, or atopic dermatitis, is a common skin condition characterized by patches of dry, red, and itchy skin. The disorder usually presents early in childhood with most cases being diagnosed by the age of 5 years. Infantile eczema most often affects the face, especially the cheeks. Many cases resolve during childhood; however, some patients can suffer from the condition throughout their life. Teenagers and adults are most often affected on the elbows and knees; however, dry scaly patches can appear anywhere on the body or face. Atopic dermatitis tends to run in families and is associated with other conditions such as asthma and allergies. The cause of eczema is not known. The disease affects between 10% to 12% of children and approximately 1% of adults.

Treatment

There is no cure for atopic dermatitis and treatment is aimed at controlling symptoms and complications. Appropriate skin care is very important. Bathing should be limited to once daily and the use of mild moisturizing cleansers is recommended. Moisturizers should be applied immediately after bathing. Itching can be treated with oatmeal (Aveeno®) or baking soda baths. Severe itching that is not relieved with appropriate baths can be treated with oral antihistamines or tricyclic antidepressants. Both oral and topical corticosteroids are used in the treatment of atopic dermatitis with oral steroids being reserved for only the most severe cases. The lowest potency topical steroids that are effective should be used to minimize side effects. Antibiotics are used to treat infectious complications. Other therapies sometimes used for severe and difficult to treat cases of eczema include phototherapy with ultraviolet A (UVA) and/or ultraviolet B (UVB) light, leukotriene inhibitors, immunosuppressants, and antineoplastics.

Review Video: Eczema
Visit mometrix.com/academy and enter code: 194210

Anaphylaxis

Anaphylaxis is a term used to describe a rapidly developing, often severe, systemic allergic reaction. An anaphylactic reaction occurs when an individual is sensitized to an allergen and then re-exposed later. Common allergens include insect bites, foods, drugs, and latex. Symptoms usually begin within thirty minutes of exposure and can include urticaria (hives), itching, generalized edema, wheezing, and difficulty breathing. Diagnosis must be made quickly and is usually based on the history and physical exam. Treatment must be initiated immediately. First priority is given to stabilizing the patient and the airway, breathing, and circulation (ABC's). The allergen should be removed, if possible. Immediate administration of intramuscular (IM) epinephrine is often required. Drug therapy may also include antihistamines, corticosteroids, and inhaled beta-agonists. Severe cases require endotracheal intubation, mechanical ventilation, and intravenous (IV) administration of epinephrine.

Human immunodeficiency virus/acquired immunodeficiency syndrome

The first cases of AIDS were described in a group of homosexual men in the United States in 1981. In 1984, it was discovered that AIDS was caused by the human retrovirus HIV. In 1985, the FDA approved the first antibody test for HIV. The number of AIDS cases has grown exponentially. It is estimated that there are currently over 42 million people living with HIV/AIDS and that by the year 2010, the number will increase by 50 to 75 million. There are approximately one million cases of

HIV/AIDS in the United States. The disease disproportionately affects minority communities. Risk factors for HIV infection include unprotected sexual intercourse, especially with multiple partners or someone who is HIV positive, IV drug abuse, a history of a blood transfusion or receiving blood products before 1985, and accidental needle sticks.

Current treatment

There is currently no cure for AIDS. Treatment goals include suppressing the viral load, and delaying immunosuppression and symptoms for as long as possible. The current treatment approach is known as highly active antiretroviral therapy (HAART). This regimen aims to reduce a patient's level of HIV as much as possible, ideally to an undetectable level. Treatment generally begins as soon as a patient is symptomatic or has a CD4 count less than 200 to 350 cells/mm^3. Treatment includes a combination of antiretroviral drugs. There are six different classes of antiretroviral drugs: nucleoside analogue reverse transcriptase inhibitors (NRTIs), protease inhibitors (PIs), non-nucleoside reverse transcriptase inhibitors (NNRTIs), nucleotide reverses transcriptase inhibitors (NtRTIs), fusion inhibitors, and integrase inhibitors. A typical treatment regimen will consist of three different drugs. Treatment also involves prophylaxis against opportunistic infection in patients with low CD4 cell counts.

Post-exposure prophylaxis

The goal of post-exposure prophylaxis is to reduce the chance of HIV infection in an individual following a potential exposure. Post-exposure prophylaxis is generally initiated after an occupational exposure or following unprotected sexual intercourse with a potentially HIV positive individual. The specific regimen depends on the type of exposure, but usually involves taking two or more antiretroviral medications for a period of four weeks. Prophylaxis must be initiated as soon as possible after the exposure. The potential benefits of post-exposure prophylaxis must be weighed against the possibility of significant side effects of the medications. Issues of compliance with the regimen and increasing HIV drug resistance as are also of concern.

Review Video: Immunomodulators and Immunosuppressive Agents
Visit mometrix.com/academy and enter code: 666131

Systemic lupus erythematosus

Systemic lupus erythematosus (SLE), or lupus, is an autoimmune disorder characterized by chronic inflammation of body tissues. The etiology cause is unknown. Certain drugs can cause a lupus like syndrome. Procainamide and hydralazine are the drugs most commonly associated with the disease. Lupus is most commonly diagnosed in women of childbearing age, but both sexes and all ages can be affected. Presenting symptoms may include the following:

- Malar rash – classic butterfly rash.
- Photosensitivity.
- Arthritis – usually affects the small joints of the hands, wrists, and feet.
- Myositis – muscle pain and weakness.
- Vasculitis.

Diagnosis and treatment

The diagnosis is made by clinical symptoms as well as serologic tests. Immunologic abnormalities, including a positive antinuclear antibody (ANA), antibodies to native deoxyribonucleic acid (DNA), anti-Smith antibodies, and antiphospholipid antibodies are all suggestive of a lupus diagnosis.

There is no cure for lupus. Treatment of lupus involves alleviating symptoms and preventing complications. Drugs used for treatment include nonsteroidal anti-inflammatory agents, corticosteroids, certain antimalarial drugs, and immunosuppressive agents. Complications include damage to vital organs such as the kidneys, lungs, central nervous system, and joints. Kidney failure is the most common cause of death in lupus patients.

Leading Causes of Death in US.
(1) Heart Dz
(2) CA
(3) Accidents
(4) Chronic lower Respiratory Dz
(5) Stroke
(6) Alzheimer's
(7) DM

Pulmonary

Asthma

Asthma is a chronic respiratory disease characterized by inflammation and constriction of the lower airways. Asthma is extremely common, affecting approximately 5% of the population in the United States. Risk factors for developing asthma include a family history, exposure to secondhand smoke, exposure to air pollution, and a history of frequent respiratory infections as a child. The cause of asthma is not known. Patients present with repeated episodes of shortness of breath, cough, and wheezing. Symptoms may be exacerbated by change in weather, exercise, viral respiratory infection, and exposure to allergens. Physical exam may be normal between episodes of asthma. During a bout of asthma, physical exam findings include wheezing, prolonged expiratory phase, and signs of respiratory distress. A chest x-ray may show hyperinflation. The diagnosis can be confirmed by spirometry performed before and after administration of a bronchodilator.

Management

The treatment regimen for asthma is depends on the severity of the disease. Mild intermittent asthma, defined as having symptoms less than two times per week, is generally treated with a short-acting beta-2 agonist inhaler on an as needed basis. Other options include an anticholinergic inhaler and a brief course of oral steroids to treat exacerbations. Mild persistent symptoms (more than two times a week) and moderate persistent symptoms (daily symptoms that occasionally affect activity) are generally treated with a daily prophylactic regimen. Options include inhaled corticosteroids, long- acting beta-2 agonists, leukotriene modifiers, and cromolyn inhalers. Severe persistent asthma is defined as daily symptoms that limit activity, and frequent exacerbations. All of the above medications can be used, as well as chronic oral corticosteroids. Treatment should also include asthma education and identification and avoidance of asthma triggers. Asthmatics require frequent follow-up.

Review Video: Asthma and Allergens
Visit mometrix.com/academy and enter code: 799141

Bronchiectasis

Bronchiectasis is a disorder characterized by an abnormal and irreversible dilation of the bronchi. The most common cause of bronchiectasis is cystic fibrosis. Other causes include immune deficiency disorders, tumors, HIV, and inhaled toxins. Presenting symptoms include a chronic cough that often produces purulent sputum, shortness of breath, wheezing, and hemoptysis. Hemoptysis is found in 50 to 70% of bronchiectasis cases. Physical exam will often be significant for an abnormal lung exam with crackles, rhonchi, and wheezing present. The patient may also have signs of chronic hypoxia, such as clubbing. Workup should include chest x-ray, CT scan, pulmonary function tests, and possible sweat testing to rule out cystic fibrosis. Treatment options include chest physiotherapy, mucolytics (DNAse), antibiotics, bronchodilators, and surgical resection.

Chronic obstructive pulmonary disease

Chronic obstructive pulmonary disease is a term that describes a group of lung disorders characterized by irreversible obstruction to airflow. Chronic bronchitis and emphysema are types of COPD. In COPD, the ability to exhale is limited, leading to air trapping and damage to lung tissue. Chronic obstructive pulmonary disease is very common; it is the fourth leading cause of death in the United States today. Risk factors for developing COPD include smoking, exposure to toxic fumes, age, and some genetic disorders like alpha-1-antitrypsin deficiency. Patients present with a chronic cough that often produces sputum, shortness of breath, exercise intolerance, and frequent respiratory infections. Pulmonary function tests, chest x-ray, arterial blood gas, and CT scan are all helpful in making the diagnosis. Treatment should include smoking cessation, pulmonary physiotherapy, and oxygen if the patient is hypoxic. Medical treatments include inhaled anticholinergics and beta agonists, antibiotics and corticosteroids. All patients should be immunized against influenza and *Pneumococcus*.

Interstitial lung disease

Interstitial lung disease refers to a group of disorders (>200), all characterized by parenchymal lung abnormalities. Interstitial lung disease can be divided into inflammatory disorders and granulomatous diseases. Examples of interstitial lung disease include idiopathic pulmonary fibrosis, sarcoidosis, Wegner's granulomatosis, bronchiolitis obliterans, Langerhans cell histiocytosis, hypersensitivity pneumonitis, and certain connective tissue disorders and autoimmune diseases. Risk factors for developing ILD include smoking, toxin exposure, and chronic exposure to high concentrations of oxygen, radiation, and chemotherapy. Patients present with shortness of breath and exercise intolerance. They may also have fatigue and weight loss. Symptoms tend to progress slowly. The diagnosis is made by clinical history, chest x-ray, CT scan, pulmonary function tests, bronchoscopy, and biopsy. A sweat chloride test should be performed to rule out cystic fibrosis. Treatment should address the underlying cause. Management can also include chest physiotherapy, immunosuppressive drugs, corticosteroids, and oxygen. Lung transplantation is sometimes and an option for severe cases.

Pleural effusion

Pleural effusion is defined as the accumulation of excess fluid in the pleural cavity. Pleural effusions can be transudative or exudative. Transudative pleural effusions result from a systemic cause that causes a disruption in the normal balance of production and absorption of pleural fluid. Diseases that can cause transudative pleural effusions are congestive heart failure, cirrhosis, pulmonary embolism, and nephritic syndrome. Exudative effusions are due to a local factor leading to either increased production or decreased lymphatic clearing of fluid. Pneumonia and cancer can cause exudative pleural effusions. Patients usually present with shortness of breath and pleuritic chest pain. Physical exam may be significant for decreased breath sounds and dullness to percussion in the area of the effusion. Diagnosis can be confirmed by chest x-ray. Pleural fluid should be obtained by thoracentesis and sent for protein, glucose, cell count, gram stain, and culture. Treatment involves addressing the underlying cause and chest tube placement for drainage in appropriate cases.

Pneumothorax

A pneumothorax occurs when there is an accumulation of air in the pleural space leading to partial or total collapse of a lung. Risk factors for developing a pneumothorax include smoking, chronic lung disease, a history of a previous pneumothorax, and being male. A pneumothorax can be spontaneous or secondary to an underlying disease or trauma. A tension pneumothorax occurs when the pressure in the pleural space is greater than atmospheric pressure. Patients present with sudden onset of chest pain and shortness of breath. If a tension pneumothorax is present, patients may be tachycardic and hypotensive. The diagnosis is confirmed with a chest x-ray. Treatment options include observation if the pneumothorax is small (<20% of the lung), needle aspiration and chest tube placement. The underlying cause of the pneumothorax must be treated.

Pulmonary embolism

A pulmonary embolism occurs when there is a blockage in the pulmonary artery or one of its branches. Risk factors for developing a pulmonary embolism include inactivity or periods of prolonged bed rest, smoking, estrogen supplementation, pregnancy and childbirth, and anything that causes a hypercoagulable state. Patients usually present with sudden onset of shortness of breath, chest pain, cough, and sometimes blood-streaked sputum. Workup should include D-dimer which is positive in >90% of patients with a pulmonary emboli, arterial blood gas, ECG, and chest x-ray. The chest x-ray is often normal or may show Westermarck's sign (a lucent area) or Hampton's hump (a wedge-shaped opacity that points towards the hilus). Diagnosis may also include spiral CT, V/Q scan, and pulmonary angiography. Treatment usually includes initial anticoagulation with heparin followed by warfarin. Embolectomy and thrombolysis are rarely used. Complications include pulmonary hypertension and cor pulmonale. Approximately one third of patients with pulmonary embolism die.

Sarcoidosis

Sarcoidosis is an immune system disorder characterized by the accumulation of granulomas (inflammatory nodules) in various organs of the body. The most commonly affected organs include the lung, lymph nodes, skin, eye, and liver. Sarcoidosis is more common in black people and women, and typically has its onset between the ages of 20 to 40 years. Symptoms of sarcoidosis vary depending on the extent and location of the disease. Many patients are asymptomatic. If the lungs are involved, patients may present with a history of a persistent, dry cough, shortness of breath, and chest pain. Patients may also have fever, weight loss, and skin lesions (erythema nodosum). The diagnosis is suggested by history and physical exam findings. The diagnosis is usually confirmed with bronchoscopy and transbronchial biopsy. The main treatment is corticosteroids. Methotrexate is also used.

Lung cancer

Lung cancer is the leading cause of cancer deaths in both men and women in the United States. Lung cancer will affect 1 in 13 men and 1 in 16 women over their lifetime. Smoking is by far the greatest risk factor and is estimated to account for close to 90% of lung cancers. Other risk factors include exposure to asbestos, radon, and secondhand smoke. Lung cancers are grouped histologically into small cell lung cancer (SCLC) and non-small cell lung cancer (NSCLC). Non-small cell lung cancers include squamous cell carcinoma, adenocarcinoma, and large cell carcinoma. Common presenting symptoms include chronic cough, change in the quality of a smoker's cough, chest pain, shortness of breath, poor appetite, and weight loss. The diagnosis is made by chest x-ray, sputum cytology, CT scan, and biopsy, via either bronchoscopy, or mediastinoscopy or an open surgical procedure.

Staging and treatment

Once lung cancer is diagnosed, staging needs to be performed. This is usually accomplished with MRI, PET scan, and bone scans. For non-small cell lung cancer, the staging is as follows: Stage I is a cancer that has not spread to the lymph nodes. A stage II cancer has spread to neighboring lymph nodes or the chest wall. Stage IIIA is defined as cancer that has spread to mediastinal lymph nodes and in stage IIIB it has spread to local organs within the chest cavity. Stage IV is distant spread of the disease. Small cell lung cancer is staged as either limited (meaning cancer is confined to one lung and local lymph nodes) or extensive (which involves both lungs and distant spread). Small cell lung cancers are generally not treated surgically. Chemotherapy and radiation are options. Non-small cell lung cancers that are stage I, II or IIIA are generally treated with surgery sometimes followed by chemotherapy and radiation. Stage IIIB and IV are not generally amenable to surgical treatment. Chemotherapy is an option, sometimes combined with radiation. The prognosis depends on the cell type and stage. The overall five-year survival is 15%.

Cardiovascular Disease

Hypertension

Hypertension is defined as a systolic blood pressure (BP) >140 mm Hg or a diastolic blood pressure >90 mm Hg measured on at least three separate occasions in adults. Values for children vary with height, gender, and age. The degree of hypertension can be defined as follows:

- Prehypertension – systolic BP 120 to 139 mm Hg or diastolic BP 80 to 89 mm Hg.
- Stage 1 hypertension – systolic BP 140 to 159 mm Hg or diastolic BP 90 to 99 mm Hg.
- Stage 2 hypertension – systolic BP >160 mm Hg or diastolic BP >100 mm Hg.

There are two classifications of hypertension. Primary or essential hypertension has no obvious etiology. Approximately 90% to 95% of hypertension is primary. Secondary hypertension is the result of some underlying condition. A thorough workup must be performed to rule out an underlying cause of hypertension. Measuring blood pressure is one of the most important parts of the physical exam and should be performed at every visit beginning in childhood.

Review Video: Hypertension
Visit mometrix.com/academy and enter code: 999599

Evaluation and treatment

First, the diagnosis of hypertension must be confirmed by at least three measurements performed on separate occasions. Next, hypertension should be classified as prehypertension, stage one, or stage two. Once the diagnosis is confirmed, a complete workup must be performed to rule out an underlying cause for hypertension. This workup should include:

- Complete history and physical exam.
- Laboratory exam including: complete blood count (CBC), urine analysis (U/A), blood glucose, lipid profile, electrolytes, blood urea nitrogen (BUN), and creatinine.
- Electrocardiogram (EKG).
- Possible use of ambulatory BP monitoring to rule out "white-coat" hypertension.

Treatment regimens involve lifestyle modification, including smoking cessation, dietary changes, and weight loss. Drug therapy is not indicated for prehypertension. Stage 1 is generally treated with a single drug, often a thiazide diuretic. Stage 2 may require combination drug therapy. Possible medications include: thiazide diuretic, angiotensin converting enzyme inhibitors (ACEI), angiotensin receptor blockers (ARB), alpha or beta-blockers, or calcium channel blockers. A diastolic BP of >120 mm Hg is generally considered a hypertensive emergency and can lead to organ damage. Immediate hospitalization and aggressive treatment is indicated.

Secondary hypertension

Secondary hypertension accounts for approximately 5% to 10% of cases. There are numerous possible causes of secondary hypertension, including the following:

- Drugs, including nonsteroidal anti-inflammatory drugs (NSAIDs), corticosteroids, Cox-2 inhibitors, weight loss medications, cold medications containing pseudoephedrine, and oral contraceptives.
- Kidney disease.

- Adrenal gland disorders.
- Disorders of the thyroid or parathyroid.
- Pre-eclampsia in pregnant women.
- Coarctation of the aorta.
- Polycythemia.

A complete workup must be performed to rule out the causes of secondary hypertension. Treatment is aimed at alleviating the underlying disorder.

Hyperlipidemia

Hyperlipidemia is defined as an elevation of serum lipid levels. Diagnosis is made by performing a screening lipid profile. A fasting lipid profile is most accurate and should be routinely performed in men over 35 years of age and women over 45 years of age. Patients with other risk factors for cardiovascular disease or with a significant family history of cardiovascular disease should be screened at a younger age. A lipid profile includes the following:

- LDL cholesterol
- HDL cholesterol
- Triglycerides
- Total cholesterol
- Cholesterol/HDL ratio

Levels at which to begin treatment depend on individual patient characteristics, including gender, age, and presence of other risk factors for coronary artery disease. In general, optimal levels are considered to be:

- LDL <100 mg/dL
- HDL >60 mg/dL
- Triglycerides <150 mg/dL
- Total cholesterol <200 mg/dL
- Cholesterol/HDL ratio <4

Management

The specific lipid levels at which to begin treatment can vary depending on the patient, but the following guidelines are usually followed:

- Triglyceride level 150 to 199 (borderline): Initiate lifestyle changes, including diet, exercise regimen, and weight loss.
- Triglyceride level 200 to 499 (high): Consider drug therapy in patients with other risk factors for coronary artery disease (CAD).
- Triglyceride level >500 (very high): Initiate drug therapy in all patients.

The different classes of drugs used in the treatment of hyperlipidemia include nicotinic acid, statins, bile acid-binding resins, and fibrates. All classes are used for lowering LDL levels. Liver function tests (LFTs) must be monitored in patients on all these drugs except for the bile-acid binding resins.

Congestive heart failure

Congestive heart failure is defined as a condition in which the heart is unable to pump sufficient blood in order to meet the needs of all the body organs. Congestive heart failure is a common disorder that affects an estimated five million people in the United States. The prevalence is highest in older individuals. Causes of CHF include previous heart attack, hypertension, coronary artery disease, cardiomyopathy, congenital heart defects, valvular disease, cardiotoxic drugs, myocarditis, and endocarditis. The four stages of CHF include:

- Stage A – individuals at risk for developing CHF.
- Stage B – structural heart disease present without symptoms.
- Stage C – structural heart disease present with symptoms.
- Stage D – advanced symptoms often not responsive to medical treatment.

Diagnosis and treatment

Clinical symptoms consistent with a CHF diagnosis include: shortness of breath at rest or with exertion, chronic fatigue, and edema. Physical exam findings may show crackles present in the lungs, dependent edema, and elevated jugular venous pressure (JVP). Cardiac exam may be significant for the presence of an S3. Further work up should include chest x-ray, EKG, and echocardiogram. Chest x-ray may show evidence of an enlarged heart. Echocardiogram may show a decreased ejection fraction. Useful laboratory tests include the brain natriuretic peptide (BNP) test. Natriuretic peptide is a protein released by myocardial cells in response to stretch. It is a useful marker for the presence of CHF. Other laboratory exams that should be obtained include: CBC, electrolytes, BUN/creatinine, fasting glucose, LFTs, and thyroid function tests.

Aortic stenosis

Aortic stenosis results from an abnormal narrowing of the aortic valve. Common causes include having a congenital bicuspid aortic valve, calcification of the aortic valve associated with aging (senile calcific aortic stenosis), and rheumatic heart disease. Symptoms result when the narrowing is sufficient to impede blood flow from the left ventricle to the aorta. Classic symptoms include shortness of breath, exercise intolerance, syncope, angina, and heart failure. Sudden death may occur during strenuous exercise, which occurs in approximately 4% of patients with aortic stenosis. Cardiac exam shows a harsh mid-systolic ejection murmur loudest at the base of the heart with radiation to the neck. An S4 may be present. Diagnosis can be confirmed with echocardiography or coronary angiography. Definitive treatment is surgical and involves valve replacement with either a bioprosthetic valve or a synthetic valve. Synthetic valves require lifelong anticoagulation therapy. All patients with a diagnosis of aortic stenosis require endocarditis prophylaxis with antibiotics.

Aortic regurgitation

Aortic regurgitation is also known as aortic insufficiency. It occurs when the aortic valve does not close properly and blood flows back into the left ventricle during diastole. The most common causes of aortic regurgitation include: congenital bicuspid aortic valve, rheumatic fever, infectious endocarditis, and Marfan syndrome. Patients are often initially asymptomatic. As the disease progresses, patients develop shortness of breath and exercise intolerance. Orthopnea is a common finding. The diagnosis can be confirmed by transesophageal echocardiogram and cardiac catheterization. Medical treatment involves afterload reduction with ACE inhibitors. Definitive treatment is surgical valve replacement. Endocarditis prophylaxis with antibiotics is often indicated.

Mitral valve prolapse

Mitral valve prolapse (MVP), also known as Barlow's syndrome, is the most common of all the heart valve disorders. It is estimated to affect 5% to 10% of the population. In this disorder, the valves are abnormally thickened due to a process known as myxomatous degeneration. The thickened valve leaflets prolapse into the left atrium during systole. Most cases are idiopathic. Other causes include genetic disorders such as Marfan's syndrome, Ehlers-Danlos syndrome, adult polycystic kidney disease, and Epstein's abnormality. It can also be the result of rheumatic heart disease. Many people with MVP are asymptomatic. Symptomatic patients present with palpitations, atypical chest pain, headache, and anxiety. The typical murmur is a midsystolic click heard best at the apex. Diagnosis can be confirmed with echocardiography. Most patients require no treatment. Symptomatic patients may require treatment with beta-blockers. Aspirin and other anticoagulants are used to reduce the risk of stroke. Surgical intervention is rarely indicated.

Mitral regurgitation

Mitral regurgitation, also known as mitral incompetence or mitral insufficiency, occurs when the mitral valve is weakened, resulting in blood leakage of blood back into the left atrium during systole. Causes of mitral regurgitation include myocardial infarction, infectious endocarditis, mitral valve prolapse, and acute rheumatic fever. Presenting symptoms include signs of left-sided heart failure, such as exercise intolerance, fatigue, and shortness of breath. Atrial fibrillation can occur because of increased pressure and damage to the right atrium. The typical murmur of mitral regurgitation is a soft blowing holosystolic murmur heard best at the left sternal border. Diagnosis can be confirmed with echocardiogram. Early diagnosis and treatment is critical before heart failure and pulmonary edema develop. The definitive treatment is surgical.

Atrial fibrillation and flutter

Atrial fibrillation is the most common arrhythmia, affecting approximately two million people in the United States. The incidence increases with age. The most common problem is clot formation and stroke, which require treatment to prevent these complications. Symptoms include palpitations, fatigue, dizziness, and shortness of breath. The diagnosis is confirmed by the absence of P waves on EKG. Medical treatment includes digoxin, beta-blockers, calcium antagonists, flecainide, and procainamide. Cardioversion is indicated when medical treatment fails. Anticoagulation may be needed to prevent stroke in high-risk patients.

Atrial flutter is an arrhythmia characterized by a very rapid atrial heart rate. Atrial flutter rates are typically 250 to 300 beats per minute. It occurs when the conduction takes an abnormal pathway through the heart. The more common route is counterclockwise and isthmus-dependent, but a clockwise conduction can occur. The diagnosis is made by the EKG. In stable patients, watchful waiting is an option. Unstable patients require cardioversion.

Ventricular tachycardia and fibrillation

Ventricular tachycardia is an abnormally rapid heart rhythm (>120 beats per minute) that originates in the ventricles. It most commonly occurs in patients with a structurally abnormal heart, often following damage from a previous myocardial infarction. Ventricular tachycardia can be monomorphic or polymorphic. Patients present with palpitations, chest pain, and syncope. There is a risk of sudden death. Diagnosis is made by EKG. Unstable patients are treated with cardioversion. Stable patients can be treated with IV amiodarone.

Ventricular fibrillation is a very rapid disorganized heart rhythm. The heart is not beating effectively and therefore is not pumping blood. It must be recognized and treated immediately to prevent death. Ventricular fibrillation often occurs following a myocardial infarction. Treatment includes immediate cardiopulmonary resuscitation (CPR) and electrical defibrillation. Survivors are at high risk for repeat episodes and should be treated with antiarrhythmic drugs or surgical implantation of an automatic defibrillator.

WPW syndrome

Wolf-Parkinson-White (WPW) syndrome is a cardiac rhythm disorder that occurs when there is an aberrant conduction pathway in the heart. Conduction can be more rapid along this extra pathway, leading to pre-excitation of the ventricles. Wolf-Parkinson-White syndrome affects approximately 0.25% of the population. Patients usually present with palpitations. They may also have chest pain, shortness of breath, or fainting. The diagnosis is made by EKG, which shows the characteristic finding of a shortened PR interval, delta waves, and a wide QRS complex. Treatment is often unnecessary. Wolf-Parkinson-White syndrome can lead to supraventricular tachycardias that must be treated. If these complications are frequent, then the ablation of the aberrant tract should be considered

Cardiomyopathy

Cardiomyopathies are disorders characterized by generalized dysfunction of the myocardial cells. There are three main types of cardiomyopathy: dilated (congestive) cardiomyopathy, hypertrophic cardiomyopathy, and restrictive cardiomyopathy.

- Dilated cardiomyopathy is characterized by diffuse ventricular enlargement. The most common etiology is coronary artery disease. Patients present with signs and symptoms of heart failure. Medical treatment includes digitalis, diuretics, and vasodilators. Advance disease may require cardiac transplantation.
- Hypertrophic cardiomyopathy is characterized by an abnormal thickening of the heart muscle. The etiology is largely unknown. It can be familial. The diagnosis is made by echocardiogram. Complications include ventricular fibrillation. Medical treatment is of limited utility. Ventriculomyotomy and implantation of a defibrillator are sometimes indicated.
- Restrictive cardiomyopathy is characterized by a stiffening of the myocardium. The most common causes are sarcoidosis and amyloidosis. Patients present with symptoms of heart failure. Diagnosis is made by EKG and echocardiogram. Medical treatment is not generally effective and the prognosis is poor. Transplantation is sometimes an option.

Acute pericarditis and pericardial effusion

Acute pericarditis is the inflammation of the pericardium. The etiology is usually infectious, most often viral. Pericardial effusion is a common complication of acute pericarditis and refers to fluid accumulation in the pericardial sac. Presenting symptoms include chest pain and fever. Pain often increases with lying down. Diagnosis is made by the presence of a friction rub on physical exam, enlarged heart on chest x-ray, and the presence of diffuse ST elevations in EKG. When a pericardial effusion is present, a patient may have shortness of breath, elevated jugular venous pressure (JVP), and muffled heart sounds. Treatment includes NSAIDs, steroids, and colchicine. Pericardial effusion requires drainage.

Peripheral vascular disease

Peripheral vascular disease is a general term referring to the pathology of the peripheral vascular system. The most common disorder is peripheral atherosclerosis. Peripheral vascular disease is common and the incidence increases with ageing. Risk factors for developing PVD include smoking, diabetes, hyperlipidemia, and hypertension. Patients often present with claudication and pain in the calf that is exacerbated with exercise. Pain at rest is a sign of advanced disease. Diagnosis is made with ultrasound and angiography. Treatment includes elimination of risk factors if possible, antiplatelet drugs, and angioplasty. Severe PVD can lead to poor wound healing and gangrene requiring amputation.

Aortic aneurysm

Aortic aneurysm refers to a weakening of the wall and eventual bulging of a part of the aorta. Atherosclerosis and hypertension are the most common causes. Aortic aneurysms can occur as a complication of Marfan's syndrome. Diagnosis is difficult, as aortic aneurysms often produce no symptoms. During a physical exam, a pulsatile abdominal mass may be felt. Diagnosis can be confirmed by x-ray or ultrasound. Dissection is the major complication of aortic aneurysms and is a life-threatening emergency. Patients present with sudden onset of intense chest pain that often radiates to the back. Patients may have signs of cardiovascular collapse, including hypotension and loss of consciousness. Treatment of aortic aneurysms is intended to prevent dissection. Small aneurysms can be treated with observation. Controlling hypertension is critical. Larger aneurysms (>4 cm) may require surgical treatment. Dissection of an aortic aneurysm is a surgical emergency and the prognosis is poor.

Ischemic heart disease

Ischemic heart disease is defined as an insufficient oxygen supply to the cardiac muscle. Ischemia can lead to necrosis and myocardial infarction. Ischemic heart disease is usually caused by atherosclerosis of the coronary arteries. Risk factors for developing ischemic heart disease include smoking, hyperlipidemia, obesity, diabetes, and increased age. Symptoms of ischemic heart disease include chest pain with exertion. When ischemic heart disease progresses to myocardial infarction, patients present with substernal chest pain that often radiates to the left arm, shortness of breath, diaphoresis, nausea, and vomiting. Diagnosis is made by history, physical exam, elevated cardiac enzymes (elevated CK-MB), and EKG changes (ST elevations). Treatment of ischemic heart disease includes risk factor reduction, nitrates, beta-blockers, and calcium channel blockers.

Myocardial infarction

Myocardial infarction is a medical emergency requiring immediate hospitalization. Treatment goals include opening of the occluded coronary arteries as quickly as possible and include the use of thrombolytic agents and coronary angioplasty. If these treatments fail, coronary artery bypass graft (CABG) should be considered.

Heart murmurs

Heart murmurs are commonly heard in children during routine physical exams and many are innocent or functional murmurs. Signs that a murmur may be pathologic include the presence of cyanosis, shortness of breath, failure to thrive, chest pain, and edema. When a heart murmur is evaluated, it should be described by location, intensity, radiation, timing during the cardiac cycle, quality, and any variation with change of position of the patient. Murmurs that are grade III or louder, or occur during diastole, are more likely to be pathologic. Patients with suspicious murmurs should have an EKG, chest x-ray, and echocardiogram. All patients with pathologic murmurs should be referred to a cardiologist.

ASD

An atrial septal defect (ASD) is a congenital heart defect in which there is a connection between the right and left atria. Risk factors for having a baby with an ASD include maternal rubella infection, maternal diabetes, and exposure to certain toxins. Usually, patients are initially asymptomatic and do not become symptomatic until their twenties. Symptoms include shortness of breath, exercise intolerance, and edema. A loud systolic ejection murmur may be heard during the exam. The diagnosis is generally made by echocardiogram. Large shunts require surgical closure. Complications include pulmonary hypertension.

VSD

A ventricular septal defect (VSD) is a congenital defect in the ventricular septum. It is the most common congenital heart defect. Risk factors are the same as for ASD. Patients are usually diagnosed by the presence of a holosystolic murmur. Small shunts are usually asymptomatic and do not require treatment. Large shunts can lead to heart failure and pulmonary hypertension and need to be treated surgically.

Cyanotic congenital heart disease

There are numerous congenital heart defects that lead to cyanosis in the newborn. They include transposition of the great vessels, total anomalous pulmonary venous return, tetralogy of Fallot, truncus arteriosus; hypoplastic left heart syndrome, tricuspid and pulmonary atresia. Patients usually present with cyanosis and signs of distress shortly after birth. The diagnosis is usually made by chest x-ray, EKG, and echocardiography. If 100% oxygen does not improve PaO_2, the cause of the cyanosis is most likely a cardiac defect. If the defect is ductus-dependent, then treatment with prostaglandins is indicated to maintain a patent ductus arteriosus. Surgery is needed for most causes of cyanotic congenital heart disease.

Dermatology

Rosacea

Rosacea is an extremely common inflammatory disease of the skin. It is characterized by facial erythema, papular and pustular lesions. It generally affects adults over the age of 30 years. It is sometimes referred to as adult acne. Patients generally present with flushing, papules, pustules, and telangiectasia on the face. These symptoms are aggravated by alcohol, spicy food, hot beverages, exercise, and temperature extremes. The diagnosis is made clinically. Treatment includes avoiding exacerbation factors, oral antibiotics, topical metronidazole, and isotretinoin. Complications include rhinophyma, a buildup of tissue around the nose, and ocular rosacea. Ocular rosacea causes a burning, gritty sensation in the eyes.

Pityriasis rosea

Pityriasis rosea is a rash commonly seen in adolescents and young adults. Patients usually present with a herald patch, a 2 to 5 cm erythematous lesion often located on the trunk. The rash then spreads, forming a characteristic "Christmas tree" pattern. It often accompanies or follows a viral upper respiratory infection. It can sometimes cause severe itching. Pityriasis rosea is a benign self-limited condition that generally requires no treatment. If itching is a problem, topical corticosteroids can be used.

Seborrheic dermatitis

Seborrheic dermatitis is a common chronic inflammatory condition that affects the scalp and skin. It can be seen in all ages. When it affects the scalp of an infant, it is known as cradle cap. The etiology is not known, but hypothesized to be caused by the fungus Malassezia furfur. It is a chronic condition. It may be exacerbated by fatigue, stress, and change of season. Patients present with patches of greasy yellow or white scales on the scalp or face. It can also be seen in skin folds. The diagnosis is generally made clinically. The scalp is treated with medicated shampoos containing coal tar, selenium sulfide, salicylic acid, pyrithione zinc, or ketoconazole. Skin lesions are treated with topical steroids or ketoconazole.

Psoriasis

Psoriasis is a chronic inflammatory skin disorder characterized by excessive and rapid skin cell production. The cause of psoriasis is unknown, but hypothesized to be immune-mediated. Exacerbating factors include infection, skin injury, stress, cold weather, smoking, alcohol, and certain medications. Human immunodeficiency virus positive individuals are at risk for severe psoriasis. Patients usually present with erythematous patches covered by silver scales. The skin is sometimes dry and cracked. Koebner's phenomenon refers to the occurrence of psoriasis at the site of trauma. Guttate psoriasis is a form of the disease often seen in younger people following a strep infection. The nails can be affected, which leads to pitting, abnormal growth, and discoloration. The diagnosis is made clinically. Treatment options include topical steroids, vitamin D analogues, and retinoids. Severe disease can be treated with phototherapy, oral retinoids, methotrexate, or cyclosporin.

Lichen planus

Lichen planus is an inflammatory disease of the skin that affects the mucous membranes, limbs, and genitalia. It usually affects adults 30 to 60 years of age. The cause is unknown. The classic skin lesions are violaceous violet papules a few millimeters in diameter. They are usually pruritic. Wickman's striae is a term to describe a surface network of white lines that are sometimes present on the skin lesions. It is usually self-limited and requires no treatment. Recurrences are common.

Cellulitis

Cellulitis is a bacterial infection of the skin. Cellulitis occurs in all age groups. People at increased risk include the elderly, immunosuppressed, diabetics, and obese individuals. Patients generally present with the affected area of the skin appearing erythematous, swollen, tender, and warm to the touch (rubor, calor, tumor, and dolor). Patients may also have fever and chills. The most common pathogens responsible for cellulitis are *Staphylococcus aureus* and streptococcal species. *Hemophilus influenzae* is seen in children. Animal bites typically cause *Pasteurella multocida* cellulitis. The workup should include a CBC, blood culture, and a wound culture if possible. Treatment is with antibiotics. Oral treatment is appropriate, but if a patient does not respond, then IV therapy may be indicated. A first generation cephalosporin or penicillinase-resistant penicillin are the typical first line drugs.

Impetigo

Impetigo is a common superficial skin infection caused by *Staphylococcus aureus* or group A streptococcus. It can affect any age group, but is commonly seen in young children. The skin lesions of impetigo typically start as pustules that easily rupture and form the classic "honey-crusted" appearance. Impetigo can be contracted from close contact with an infected individual. The diagnosis is made clinically and treatment is good hygiene along with either topical or oral antibiotics. Usually, impetigo is easily treated. Possible complications include post-strep glomerulonephritis, cellulitis, and invasive methicillin-resistant *Staphylococcus aureus* (MRSA) infection.

Erysipelas

Erysipelas is an acute skin infection caused by *Streptococcus pyogenes*. It is usually seen in the very young, the elderly, or immunocompromised patients. Patients present with fever, shaking, chills, and a rash that is well demarcated, erythematous, firm, and tender. Lymphangitic streaking may be present. Complications include bacteremia and sepsis. Treatment is with IV antibiotics.

Fungal skin infections

<u>Tinea versicolor</u>

Tinea versicolor is a common chronic fungal infection of the skin that causes hyper- or hypopigmented lesions. It is most often seen in adolescents and young adults and is more common in warm humid climates. Patients present with discolored macular lesions that may be itchy. The diagnosis is made by KOH prep, which will show budding hyphae. Treatment is with topical antifungal creams. Occasionally, systemic antifungals are needed.

<u>Candidiasis</u>

Candidiasis, commonly known as yeast infection, can cause a wide variety of infections including superficial skin infections, oral thrush, and vaginitis. Risk factors for developing *Candida* infections include obesity, diabetes, steroid, and antibiotic use. The typical rash involves erythematous lesions of varying sizes and satellite lesions. Vesicular and pustular lesions are usually present. Diagnosis is made by KOH prep, which shows pseudohyphae. Treatment is with topical antifungals.

Parasitic skin infections

Scabies

Scabies is an intensely pruritic skin infection cause by the mite *Sarcoptes scabiei*. The disease is spread by close physical contact with an infected individual. All ages are affected. The typical presentation is an erythematous rash with tracks and burrows. It can often appear excoriated from scratching. It is usually seen between the fingers, in the axillae, on the soles of the feet, and in the genital area. The diagnosis is made clinically. Skin scrapings may reveal the presence of mites or their eggs. Treatment options include permethrin and crotamiton. It is sometimes necessary to treat family members in order to eradicate the disease.

Pediculosis

Pediculosis is a skin infection from lice. The same organism causes head lice. Patients are often asymptomatic. The diagnosis is made by visualizing the lice. Head lice can be visualized using a Wood's lamp, which makes nits appear pale blue in color. Treatment is with permethrin shampoo, malathion shampoo, or lindane (cream, lotion, or shampoo).

Stevens-Johnson syndrome

Stevens-Johnson syndrome, or erythema multiforme major, is a severe inflammatory condition of the skin thought to be caused by a drug reaction. The medications thought to be responsible for most cases of Stevens-Johnson syndrome are sulfa drugs, phenytoin, carbamazepine, lamotrigine, allopurinol, and the NSAIDs. Stevens-Johnson syndrome can also follow an infection such as herpes, influenza, or hepatitis. The patient presents with tongue and facial swelling, mucosal erosions (especially in the mouth), skin sloughing, diffuse hives, and target lesions. The diagnosis is generally based on the history and physical exam. Treatment includes stopping any offending medication and supportive care with pain medication, IV fluids, and local skin care. In severe cases, patients may require nasogastric feeding and skin grafting. Complications include cellulitis and sepsis.

Toxic epidermal necrolysis

Toxic epidermal necrolysis is a severe, life-threatening inflammatory skin condition that is generally felt to be an allergic reaction to a medication. The medications felt to be most often responsible for toxic-epidermal necrolysis are sulfa drugs, phenytoin, carbamazepine, lamotrigine, allopurinol, and NSAIDs. Patients present with severe swelling and mucosal erosions in the mouth, nose, and eyes. They have a diffuse erythematous rash with target lesions. The rash often coalesces and rapidly progresses to necrosis and peeling. Patients may have a positive Nikolsky's sign (spread of blisters upon application of pressure to the skin). The diagnosis is made clinically. Treatment includes supportive care and discontinuing use of offending. Patients often require admission to a burn unit. Intravenous immunoglobulin may be helpful. The mortality is 30-40%.

Melanoma

Melanoma is a malignant tumor of melanocytes. Risk factors for developing melanoma include a history of excessive sun exposure and sunburn, fair skin, dysplastic moles, positive family history, and being immunocompromised. Melanomas can appear anywhere, but most often occur on sun-exposed areas such as the back, face, and extremities. Patients present with a history of a change in an existing mole or development of new lesions. Characteristics of moles that should arouse suspicion of melanoma include: asymmetry, irregular borders, a change in the color or irregularity of color, diameter of >¼ inch, and history of the mole changing over time. A history of bleeding from the mole may also indicate melanoma. The diagnosis is made by biopsy. Treatment is surgery, chemotherapy, and radiation. Prognosis is dependent on the stage of disease at diagnosis. If there is distant spread, the five-year survival is about 10%.

Basal cell carcinoma

Basal cell carcinoma is the most common form of skin cancer, accounting for about 80%. Risk factors for developing basal cell carcinoma include having fair skin, a family history of the disease, and history of sun exposure. The most common location is the head and neck, but they can occur anywhere. It is more common in men. Basal cell carcinomas usually appear as pearly white, waxy papular lesions. Diagnosis is made by biopsy and treatment is excision. Metastatic spread is extremely rare.

Actinic keratosis

Actinic keratosis is a slow growing skin lesion that is considered premalignant for squamous cell carcinoma. They appear as flat or slightly raised scaly lesions that vary in color. Treatment is cryotherapy. Topical 5-fluorouracil and imiquimod are also used.

Squamous cell carcinoma

Squamous cell carcinoma is the second most common skin cancer. The appearance can vary from a firm red papule to a flat, crusted, or scaly lesion. They can occur anywhere on the body. Treatment is removal using Mohs' surgery. Removal is generally curative.

Endocrinology

Diabetes

Type 1 diabetes mellitus

Type 1 diabetes, which is also sometimes referred to as juvenile onset diabetes or insulin dependent diabetes, is an autoimmune disease characterized by total destruction of the insulin producing islet cells of the pancreas. The cause of type 1 diabetes is unknown. This disease is generally diagnosed in children or young adults (average age at diagnosis is 14 years). Presenting symptoms include weight loss and dehydration as well as the "3 P's": polyuria, polydipsia, and polyphagia. Patients may present in diabetic ketoacidosis (DKA). Diagnosis is made by serum glucose level or a glucose tolerance test. A random glucose level of >200 mg/dL or a fasting level of >126 mg/dL is diagnostic. Patients must be treated with insulin. Education regarding tight management of glucose levels is critical to avoid complications. Occasionally, patients undergo pancreas transplantation.

Review Video: Diabetes and Insulin
Visit mometrix.com/academy and enter code: 666371

Review Video: Diabetes Type I
Visit mometrix.com/academy and enter code: 501396

Type 2 diabetes mellitus

Type 2 diabetes mellitus, which is also known as adult onset or non-insulin dependent diabetes, is characterized by insulin resistance. Type 2 diabetes accounts for approximately 90% of diabetes mellitus cases. Risk factors for the development of type 2 diabetes include obesity, family history, race, and age. The diagnosis is more common in blacks, Hispanics, American Indians, and Asian Americans. It is also more commonly diagnosed in persons over the age of 45 years, although diagnosis in children is becoming more common. Patients present with weight loss and the "3 P's": polyuria, polydipsia, and polyphagia. Treatment involves dietary management, oral hypoglycemic agents, and insulin.

Chronic complications of diabetes

The chronic complications of diabetes can be divided into three groups: macrovascular complications, microvascular complications, and neuropathies. Macrovascular complications include coronary artery disease, which results in increased risk of myocardial infarction, stroke, and congestive heart failure. Coronary artery disease is responsible for 70% of the mortality associated with diabetes. Microvascular complications include retinopathy and nephropathy, which can result in blindness and kidney failure. Neuropathies usually affect the distal extremities and increase the patient's risk for traumatic lesions. The diabetic patient must be followed closely for the onset of complications. Yearly eye exams, kidney functions screening, and careful foot exams are critical. Chronic complications generally start to appear five or more years following diagnosis. The onset of complications can be delayed or prevented with tight control of blood glucose levels.

DKA

Diabetic ketoacidosis (DKA) is more likely to develop in patients with type 1 diabetes. Insufficient or absent insulin results in increased gluconeogenesis and ketogenesis, leading to very elevated levels of plasma glucose and ketones. This causes an osmotic diuresis that may result in severe dehydration. Risk factors for development of DKA include infection, not taking prescribed insulin, or newly diagnosed diabetes. Classic symptoms include: abdominal pain, vomiting, dehydration, altered mental status, Kussmaul respirations, and 'ketone breath' (a fruity odor due to high ketone levels). The diagnosis is made by laboratory findings, including an extremely elevated glucose and a high ion gap metabolic acidosis. Immediate therapy includes IV fluids (normal saline followed by 1/2NS; glucose should be added when serum glucose is below 250 mg/dL), insulin drip, and electrolyte replacement.

Hyperosmolar coma

In hyperosmolar coma (nonketotic hyperglycemia), patients present with extremely elevated serum glucose, often >800 mg/dL, and altered mental status. Acidosis is not present and serum pH >7.3. Treatment includes fluid and electrolyte replacement and insulin drip. Prognosis is guarded with mortality as high as 50%.

Hypoglycemia

Hypoglycemia and hypoglycemic coma are common complications of diabetes and should be considered in any patient in a comatose state of unknown etiology. Presenting symptoms include change in mental status ranging from confusion to coma, palpitations, trembling, and tachycardia. If the patient is awake, treatment includes oral administration of glucose. Comatose patients are treated with intramuscular (IM) glucagon (1 mg) or an IV infusion of 50% glucose.

Hyper-/Hypo- thyroidism

Hyperthyroidism, or thyrotoxicosis, is defined as an elevated level of circulating thyroid hormone. The most common form of thyrotoxicosis is Grave's disease. Presenting symptoms of hyperthyroidism include fatigue, weight loss, heat intolerance, anxiety, palpitations, and tremulousness. On physical exam, patients appear hyperactive and nervous. Sweating, tremors, tachycardia, hyperreflexia, and thin hair are present. Patients with Grave's disease also have exophthalmos and pretibial myxedema. The thyroid may be enlarged. The diagnosis is made by laboratory exam tests of thyroid function tests including TSH, free T3, free T4, and thyroid antibodies. A radioactive iodine uptake and scan should be performed to differentiate between Grave's disease, solitary toxic nodule, multinodular goiter, subacute thyroiditis, and exogenous hyperthyroidism. Treatment includes antithyroid medications such as propylthiouracil (PTU) and methimazole (MMI), administration of radioactive iodine, and thyroidectomy.

Hypothyroidism is defined as inadequate production of thyroid hormone. Hypothyroidism can be primary, secondary, or tertiary. Primary hypothyroidism is the most common type and it is caused by a defect in the thyroid gland leading to inadequate production of thyroid hormone. Examples of causes of primary hypothyroidism include Hashimoto's thyroiditis, iodine deficiency, and drugs such as amiodarone, lithium, interleuken-2, and alpha- interferon. Primary hypothyroidism can also occur following thyroidectomy, radioactive iodine treatment, or neck irradiation. Secondary hypothyroidism is due to pituitary failure. Tertiary hypothyroidism is due to hypothalamic failure. Presenting symptoms include weight gain, fatigue, cold intolerance, and dry skin. Classic physical findings include hoarse voice, periorbital edema, sluggish deep tendon reflexes, and an enlarged tongue. The diagnosis is confirmed by checking thyroid function tests. In primary hypothyroidism, the TSH will be elevated and free T4 is decreased. Hypothyroidism is treated with thyroid hormone replacement. Levels must be followed closely.

Review Video: 7 Symptoms of Hyperthyroidism
Visit mometrix.com/academy and enter code: 923159

Hyper-/Hypo- calcemia

Hypercalcemia is defined as an elevated serum calcium level. There are numerous causes, the most common of which are hyperparathyroidism and cancer. Clinical manifestations of hypercalcemia include fatigue, weakness, confusion, passage of renal stones, nausea, vomiting, and abdominal pain. The diagnosis is made by laboratory examination of serum calcium, parathyroid hormone (PTH), and phosphate levels. Computerized tomography scan or chest x-ray may be needed to rule out malignancy. The goal of treatment is to lower the calcium level. Possible treatments include IV fluids, calcitonin, corticosteroids, IV bisphosphonates, oral phosphate, and dialysis as a last resort. Primary hyperparathyroidism can be treated surgically. Underlying malignancy should be treated appropriately.

Hypocalcemia is an abnormally low level of serum calcium. Hypocalcemia can be caused by hypoparathyroidism, pseudohypoparathyroidism, chronic renal failure, and deficiency in vitamin D or magnesium. Other causes of hypocalcemia can also include chronic renal failure, magnesium deficiency or it can occur as a complication of chemotherapy. Certain medications including diuretics, estrogens, laxatives, and magnesium can sometimes be associated with hypocalcemia. Diagnosis is made by a low serum calcium level. It is important to check serum albumin and correct for hypoalbuminemia since approximately half of the circulating calcium is bound to albumin. Measuring the ionized, or free, calcium is the most clinically significant.

Presentation and treatment

Patients with hypocalcemia present with neuromuscular irritability, or tetany. Other findings in hypocalcemia include Chvostek's sign and Trousseau's sign. A positive Chvostek's sign is elicited by tapping on the facial nerve. This leads to an involuntary contraction of the facial muscles on the same side of the face. Trousseau's sign is elicited by inflating a blood pressure cuff above an individual's systolic blood pressure for a few minutes. A hypocalcemic patient will respond with an involuntary contraction of the wrist and meta-carpo-phalangeal (MCP) joints, hyperextension of the fingers, and flexion of the thumb. This is known as carpal spasm. Electrocardiogram may show a prolongation of the QT interval. Diagnosis is made by a low serum calcium level. It is important to check serum albumin and correct for hypoalbuminemia. Treatment involves IV calcium if severe symptoms are present. Mild cases can be treated with oral calcium.

Adrenal insufficiency

Primary adrenal insufficiency is known as Addison's disease. It occurs when the adrenal cortex fails to produce sufficient levels of cortisone. Causes of primary adrenal insufficiency include: autoimmune destruction of the adrenal cortex, tumor, hemorrhage, infections, and as a complication of certain medications. Adrenal insufficiency can be seen if patients on long-term corticosteroid therapy are withdrawn too quickly. Secondary adrenal insufficiency is due to inadequate pituitary production of adrenocorticotropic hormone (ACTH). Presenting symptoms include weakness, weight loss, nausea, vomiting, and abdominal pain. Hyperpigmentation is seen in primary adrenal insufficiency. Acute adrenal failure, also known as Addisonian crisis, is a medical emergency characterized by severe vomiting, diarrhea, hypotension, and hyperkalemia, ultimately leading to coma and death if untreated. Diagnosis is made by checking cortisol levels and by doing an ACTH stimulation test. If an elevated ACTH level is present, it is suggestive of primary disease. Treatment is cortisol replacement.

Review Video: Addison's Disease
Visit mometrix.com/academy and enter code: 813552

Paget's disease

Paget's disease is a bone disorder characterized by an increased rate of bone remodeling. Paget's disease is common and usually affects people over the age of 40 years. The etiology is unknown. Many patients are asymptomatic. Symptoms include bone and joint pain as well as fractures and deformities. Nerve impingement can occur. Laboratory exam shows an elevated level of alkaline phosphatase. X-ray examination may show increased density and size of involved bones. Affected areas will light up on bone scan. Asymptomatic patients do not require treatment. Symptomatic patients are treated with bisphosphonates or calcitonin.

Cushing's disease

Cushing's syndrome occurs as the result of an excess of cortisol and can be caused by excessive steroid therapy. Another cause is increased levels of ACTH, either from a pituitary abnormality or from another neoplasm such as small cell carcinoma of the lung and adrenal tumors. The classic cushingoid presentation is obesity, "moon face", and "buffalo hump." Patients also have fatigue, weakness, and exhibit poor healing of skin lesions. Irregular menses and glucose intolerance may also be present. Diagnosis is made by measuring morning cortisol levels and by performing an overnight dexamethasone suppression test. To help determine the etiology, ACTH levels should be checked. Computerized tomography and magnetic resonance imaging (MRI) may be needed to rule out tumors. Treatment depends on the etiology of the increased cortisol.

Syndrome of inappropriate antidiuretic hormone secretion

The syndrome of inappropriate antidiuretic hormone secretion (SIADH) results from excessively high levels of antidiuretic hormone (ADH) secretion leading to the inappropriate production of concentrated urine. This leads to hyponatremia and volume overload. There are many causes of SIADH, including tumors (small cell carcinoma of the lung in particular), central nervous system (CNS) trauma or infection, and various medications. Presenting symptoms include nausea, fatigue, and headache that can progress to lethargy and coma if untreated. The diagnosis is made by laboratory examination, which reveals hyponatremia or low plasma osmolality in the presence of concentrated urine. Management includes water restriction with gradual correction of sodium. Loop diuretics, lithium, and demeclocycline are also used sometimes.

Diabetes insipidus

Diabetes insipidus (DI) results from inadequate secretion of ADH leading to excessive production of very diluted urine. Diabetes insipidus can be central, nephrogenic, dipsogenic, or gestational. Central DI is caused by ADH deficiency resulting from a hypothalamic or pituitary problem. Nephrogenic DI is caused by a resistance to ADH in the kidney. Dipsogenic DI refers to abnormal thirst and excessive intake of water. Gestational DI is a complication of pregnancy. Patients generally present with polyuria, polydipsia, and dehydration. The diagnosis is confirmed by the presence of a high plasma osmolality and diluted urine. The diagnosis can also be made by administering a water deprivation test or vasopressin test. Treatment involves treating any underlying cause and DDAVP administration.

Hypopituitarism

Hypopituitarism is defined as a failure of the pituitary gland to produce sufficient quantities of one or more of the pituitary hormones. Etiologies include idiopathic, tumors, head trauma, CNS infections, and iatrogenic causes (e.g., post-radiation treatment). Infarction or hemorrhage, as in Sheehan's syndrome and pituitary apoplexy, are also causes. Primary and secondary empty sella syndrome can also lead to hypopituitarism. Presenting symptoms vary according to the particular hormones that are deficient. Diagnosis is made by measuring hormone levels. Treatment is aimed at correcting an underlying cause if present and hormone replacement.

Hormones secreted by pituitary gland

Anterior pituitary gland:

- Growth hormone – promotes growth.
- Thyroid-stimulation hormone (TSH) – stimulates secretion of thyroid hormones.
- Adrenocorticotropic hormone (ACTH) – stimulates secretion or glucocorticoids.
- Prolactin - stimulates milk production in post-partum women.
- Luteinizing hormone (LH) – stimulates secretion of sex steroids.
- Follicle stimulation hormone (FSH) – stimulates follicle development.

Posterior pituitary gland:

- Antidiuretic hormone – water reabsorption in the kidney.
- Oxytocin – stimulates uterine contraction during labor and milk letdown post-delivery.

Gastroenterology

Peptic ulcer disease

Peptic ulcers are eroded lesions of the mucosa of the stomach or duodenum. Most (up to 80%) peptic ulcer disease is caused by *Helicobacter pylori* infection. The majority arises in the duodenum and is benign. Stomach ulcers are more likely to be caused by a malignancy. Ulcers can also occur in the esophagus and are usually related to esophageal reflux. Other risk factors for PUD include smoking, NSAID use, and excessive alcohol use. The classic presenting symptom of duodenal ulcers is nighttime stomach pain relieved by eating. Gastric ulcers typically present with pain following a meal. Less frequently, ulcers can present with hematemesis, black tarry stools, nausea, vomiting, and weight loss. The diagnosis is made with endoscopy and *H pylori* serology. Treatment includes an antibiotic regimen to eliminate *H pylori* infection. This usually involves two antibiotics, often amoxicillin and metronidazole for two weeks. Histamine-2 blockers, proton pump inhibitors and antacids can also be used. Follow-up endoscopy should be performed to confirm healing.

Gastritis

Gastritis is inflammation of the mucosal lining of the stomach. Gastritis can be acute or chronic. Causes include *H pylori* infection, chronic use of NSAIDs, excessive alcohol consumption, bile reflux, and other chronic illnesses. Patients typically present with dyspepsia, nausea, vomiting, weight loss, and a full or bloated feeling. Patients sometimes present with gastrointestinal bleeding. The diagnosis is usually made clinically, but can include *H pylori* testing and endoscopy. Treatment includes antacids, H2 blockers, proton pump inhibitors, and antibiotics to eradicate *H pylori.*

Esophageal dysphagia

Esophageal dysphagia is difficulty swallowing. It is distinct from odynophagia, which is defined as painful swallowing. Causes include mechanical obstruction from strictures, tumors or foreign bodies, motility disorders including achalasia, and spasm of the esophagus. Patients present with difficulty swallowing, choking or coughing during eating, weight loss and pneumonias. The diagnosis can be made with endoscopy, barium swallow, and monometric studies of the esophagus. Treatment approach depends on the underlying cause and may include occupational therapy to aid in swallowing, acid blocking medications, and surgery to remove obstructions.

Gastroesophageal reflux disease

Gastroesophageal reflux disease (GERD) is a condition in which stomach contents flow back up into the esophagus. It is caused by a failure of the normal anti-reflux mechanisms. Inciting factors include smoking, alcohol, consuming large meals, and assuming a supine position shortly after meals. Symptoms of GE reflux are common during pregnancy. Presenting symptoms include heartburn and chest pain often made worse by lying down. Patients may regurgitate sour-tasting material. Patients can also have hoarseness, sore throat, coughing, and wheezing. The diagnosis is generally based on clinical history. Useful tests include endoscopy and twenty-four hour esophageal pH probe monitoring. Treatment includes antacids, H2 blockers, proton pump inhibitors, and prokinetic medications. In cases of mechanical problems, surgery is sometimes needed. Nissen fundoplication is a surgical procedure to tighten the lower esophageal sphincter.

Lifestyle management is also indicated and includes eating more frequent, smaller meals, avoiding reflux-inducing foods, elevating the head of the bed, and cessation of smoking and alcohol use.

Review Video: Peptic Ulcers and GERD
Visit mometrix.com/academy and enter code: 184332

Diarrhea

Acute diarrhea

Acute diarrhea is the increased output of watery stool for less than two weeks duration. The most common causes are infectious, including viral, bacterial, and parasitic pathogens. Other causes include complications from certain medications, toxins, inflammatory bowel disease, and diverticulitis. The workup for acute diarrhea involves sending stool samples for culture (both bacterial and viral), fecal leukocytes, and ova and parasites (O&P). Stool should be checked for *Clostridium difficile* antigen in patients with a recent history of antibiotic use. Endoscopy may be needed to rule out inflammatory bowel disease. Most cases of acute diarrhea are self-limited and do not require treatment. Patients must be given adequate fluid and electrolyte replacement and treated for dehydration if necessary. Antibiotic treatment is indicated for certain cases of bacterial diarrhea, including invasive *Salmonella*, *Shigella*, *Campylobacter*, and *Yersinia* septicemia. Diarrhea due to parasites usually requires treatment.

Chronic diarrhea

Chronic diarrhea is the increased output of watery stool for more than two weeks duration. Chronic diarrhea has both infectious and non-infectious causes. Infectious causes include viruses, bacteria, and parasites. Non-infectious causes include inflammatory bowel disease, malabsorption syndromes, food allergies, and use of certain medications. Diagnosis should follow an organized approach dependent on the patient's history and physical exam. Diagnostic tests may include stool for culture, ova and parasite exam, and fecal leukocytes. Endoscopy may be considered to rule out inflammatory bowel disease. Studies for malabsorption syndromes include fecal pH, stool-reducing substances, breath hydrogen test, and stool for fecal fat. Treatment will depend on the cause of the chronic diarrhea.

Lactose intolerance

Lactose intolerance is the inability to completely digest lactose due to a deficiency of the enzyme lactase. Lactose intolerance is very common and may be present from birth. It has a particularly high prevalence in people of East Asian and Native American descent. Lactose intolerance can develop as the result of aging and decreased lactose production. Lactose intolerance can also result from bowel injury following gastroenteritis or may be due to inflammatory bowel disease. Patients present with abdominal pain, gas, cramps, and diarrhea following ingestion of dairy products. The diagnosis is confirmed by a lactose tolerance test, hydrogen breath test, or stool acidity test. Treatment includes reducing or eliminating dairy products from the diet, taking lactase tablets, and calcium and vitamin supplementation.

Review Video: Lactose Intolerance
Visit mometrix.com/academy and enter code: 672651

Celiac disease

Celiac disease is an autoimmune disease that occurs in genetically predisposed individuals. Damage to the mucosa of the small intestine leads to an inability to properly digest gluten. The disease is triggered by a reaction to the gliden protein found in gluten. This condition has also been called celiac sprue, or gluten-sensitive enteropathy. Patients present with varied and non-specific symptoms, including diarrhea, cramps, weight loss and failure to thrive in children. Complications include malnutrition, lactose intolerance, and certain cancers, particularly intestinal lymphoma and colon cancer. Diagnosis is made by elevation of antiendomysial IgA and anti-tissue transglutaminase IgA, and by small intestinal biopsy. Treatment is the avoidance of gluten in the diet.

Ulcerative colitis

Ulcerative colitis is a type of inflammatory bowel disease. The cause is unknown, but there appears to be a hereditary component. It is more common in women and is typically diagnosed between the ages of 30 to 50 years. Presenting symptoms vary, but can include abdominal pain, change in bowel habits, straining, urgency, and bloating. Bloody stools are frequently present. Fulminant colitis is a rare complication in which the entire colon is affected. Patients present with copious diarrhea, dehydration, shock, and occasionally toxic megacolon and colonic rupture. Diagnosis is made by sigmoidoscopy or colonoscopy, which reveals the characteristic mucosal inflammation, erosions, and bleeding. The rectum is always involved and the disease is continuous, spreading up the colon. Treatment includes dietary measures. Medical treatment may include sulfasalazine, mesalamine, balsalazide, and corticosteroids. Colectomy is sometimes indicated for severe disease and it is curative.

Crohn's disease

Crohn's disease is a type of inflammatory bowel disease. The cause is unknown, but there appears to be a hereditary component. Presenting symptoms include abdominal pain, cramping, chronic diarrhea, fever, weight loss, and fatigue. Strictures, fistulas, and abscesses are all possible complications of Crohn's disease. Aphthous ulcers, anal fissures, perirectal abscesses, and anorectal fistulas are classic findings on physical exam. The diagnosis is made by colonoscopy, which shows transmucosal inflammation. Crohn's disease can affect any part of the GI tract and it is most often seen in the colon and small bowel. Medical treatment involves use of anti-inflammatory drugs and immunosuppressive agents. Anti-inflammatory drugs used include sulfasalazine, mesalamine, and corticosteroids. Immunosuppressive agents used include azathioprine, 6-mercaptopurine, methotrexate, and cyclosporine. Since Crohn's disease can be seen throughout the GI tract and is not continuous, surgery is not curative.

Constipation

Constipation is defined as infrequent, hard or difficult to pass bowel movements. In general, passing a bowel movement fewer than three times per week is considered abnormal. Constipation is very common and affects both sexes and all ages. There are many causes of constipation:

Acute:

- Medications such as narcotics
- Spasm of the anal sphincter
- Obstruction

Chronic:

- Inflammatory bowel disease
- Rectal abnormalities
- Endocrine abnormalities (hypothyroidism)
- Neurologic disorders (MS, spinal cord injury)
- Inadequate fluid intake
- Low fiber diet

Workup and treatment depend on the individual's history and physical exam. Most cases of constipation are benign and self-limited and are easily treated with dietary changes and stool softeners.

Cirrhosis of the liver

Cirrhosis is irreversible scarring and fibrosis of the liver. There are numerous causes, the most common of which are alcoholism and hepatitis (usually hepatitis B or C). The other causes of cirrhosis include autoimmune liver disease, nonalcoholic fatty liver disease, hemochromatosis, Wilson's disease, cystic fibrosis, biliary atresia, alpha 1-antitrypsin deficiency, and glycogen storage disease. Presenting symptoms of cirrhosis include fatigue, loss of appetite, nausea, vomiting, and abdominal pain. On physical exam, the typical findings include an enlarged firm liver, spider angiomas, jaundice, and ascites.

Workup

The workup to determine the cause of liver failure includes laboratory examinations, such as liver function tests (LFTs), CBC, and albumin. Hepatitis screening should be performed. Ultrasound, CT, and MRI imaging may be helpful to assess the extent of disease. Liver biopsy is often needed to determine the cause. Cirrhosis is generally irreversible. Treatment is aimed at halting progression and alleviating symptoms. Alcohol use should be stopped. Treatments for hepatitis include interferon and other medications. Potentially hepatotoxic drugs like acetaminophen should be stopped. Ascites can be treated with paracentesis, which usually needs to be repeated. Patients with advanced disease should be considered for liver transplantation.

Syndromes associated with liver disease

The following conditions are associated with liver disease:

- Spontaneous bacterial peritonitis (SBP) – infection of ascites fluid with gut bacteria.
- Hepatorenal syndrome – renal failure that occurs as a complication of cirrhosis.
- Hepatic encephalopathy – possibly due to elevated ammonia levels.
- Esophageal varices – grossly dilated submucosal veins of the esophagus.
- Bleeding has a mortality rate of 20%.
- Hepatopulmonary syndrome – refers to the hypoxemia that develops as a complication of chronic liver disease.

Gallstones and cholecystitis

Cholecystitis is inflammation of the gallbladder and it is the most common complication of gallstones. Cholecystitis can be acute or chronic. Acute cholecystitis is characterized by the sudden onset of severe, constant, right upper quadrant (RUQ) abdominal pain, and fever. Chronic cholecystitis is characterized by repeated bouts of biliary pain. Symptoms often follow a large fatty meal. Physical exam may be significant for RUQ tenderness, a positive Murphy's sign, jaundice, and a palpable gallbladder. The diagnosis is made by laboratory exam, showing increased bilirubin. White blood cell count and LFTs are frequently elevated. The diagnosis can be confirmed with ultrasound, HIDA scan, or cholangiography. Patients should be hospitalized, ingest nothing by mouth (NPO), and given IV fluids, antibiotics, and pain medication. Surgery is usually indicated.

Acute pancreatitis

Pancreatitis is inflammation of the pancreas. Patients with acute pancreatitis present with sudden onset of severe upper abdominal pain that radiates to the back. In addition, patients often have nausea, vomiting, and fever. Physical exam may reveal hypotension, tachycardia, and signs of shock. The abdominal exam is significant for diffuse tenderness. Pancreatic characteristics include Cullen's sign, Grey Turner's sign, ecchymosis around the umbilicus, and ecchymosis of the flanks. The most common causes are gallstones and alcohol. Other causes include certain medications (steroids, NSAIDs), post-surgery complications, infectious, idiopathic, abdominal trauma, and pancreatic cancer. Laboratory workup should include a serum amylase, which is typically significantly elevated, CBC, LFTS, serum lipase, and an arterial blood gas. Ultrasound and CT scan are helpful in making the diagnosis. Patients with acute pancreatitis require hospitalization. They should be made NPO and treated with broad-spectrum antibiotics. Most cases are self-limited. Potential complications include pancreatic necrosis, abscess, pseudocysts, ascites, and pleural effusions.

Acute GI bleed

Acute GI bleeding is a medical emergency. Bleeding may arise from the upper or lower GI tracts. Upper GI bleeding usually presents with hematemesis and melena. Lower GI bleeds can present with blood-streaked stools if the bleed is distal (rectosigmoid to anus), maroon colored stools for bleeds in the right colon or small intestine, and melena if the bleed is proximal to the ligament of Treitz. Massive bleeding can present with hematochezia. Immediate management includes resuscitation and stabilization of the patient. Patients should be made NPO, aggressive IV rehydration should be started, and a nasogastric (NG) tube should be inserted. Blood work should include a CBC, type and cross-match. The location of the bleed should be determined by history, exam findings, and possibly endoscopy, colonoscopy or nuclear bleeding scan. Once the source is determined, appropriate therapy should be initiated to stop the bleed.

Cancer

Esophageal cancer

Esophageal cancer is typically seen in men over the age of 50 years. Risk factors for developing esophageal cancer include excessive alcohol use, tobacco use, and Barrett's esophagus (chronic changes due to GE reflux). Esophageal cancer is sometimes associated with achalasia, esophageal webs, or tylosis. Patients usually present with difficulty swallowing, weight loss, and voice hoarseness. The diagnosis is confirmed by upper endoscopy and biopsy. Surgery is sometimes curative for early-stage disease. Late-stage disease cannot be treated surgically. Chemotherapy and radiation can be palliative in advanced cases.

Gastric cancer

Gastric cancer is relatively uncommon in the United States; the prevalence is higher in other parts of the world. Development of gastric cancer is associated with chronic *H pylori* infection and chronic gastritis. The most common cell type is adenocarcinoma and it is more common in men over the age of 40 years. Symptoms are often absent early in the disease. Eventually, patients develop abdominal pain, early satiety, weight loss and black, tarry stools. The diagnosis is made by endoscopy and biopsy. Computerized tomography scan is needed for staging of the disease. Surgery is an option for early stage disease. Advanced disease can be treated with palliative surgery and chemotherapy. The prognosis is poor, with an average five-year survival rate of 15%.

Colorectal cancer

Colorectal cancer is the second most common cancer in the United States, affecting both men and women. The diagnosis is typically made after the age of 40 years and risk factors include a positive family history, history of polyps or inflammatory bowel disease, and consuming a diet high in fat and red meat. All patients should begin screening for colon cancer by colonoscopy at age 50 years. Patients with risk factors should begin screening at age 40 years. Patients should be screened every five years. If polyps are found during screening, colonoscopy should be repeated every three years. The most common presenting symptom is blood in the stool. The diagnosis is made by colonoscopy. Carcinoembryonic antigen (CEA) levels can be used as a marker of disease. Treatment involves surgery, radiation, and chemotherapy. The prognosis is highly dependent on the stage of disease at diagnosis.

Hepatocellular carcinoma

Hepatocellular carcinoma is a primary cancer of the liver. It is usually associated with chronic cirrhosis due to hepatitis infection or alcoholic liver disease. Patients usually present with weight loss and generalized weakness. Hepatomegaly with or without a palpable mass may be present on physical exam. The diagnosis is made by liver biopsy. Treatment options depend on the stage of the disease and include: liver transplantation, surgical resection, chemoembolization, ethanol injection, and radiofrequency ablation. Screening methods are not routinely agreed. Patients with risk factors may be screened with ultrasound and alpha-fetoprotein (AFP) level monitoring. The prognosis is generally poor.

Pancreatic cancer

Pancreatic cancer is a primary tumor of the pancreas. Risk factors include obesity, smoking, history of pancreatitis, and a family history of pancreatic cancer. Pancreatic cancer is often asymptomatic until late in the disease. Symptoms include upper abdominal pain, jaundice, loss of appetite, and weight loss. Physical exam may reveal an epigastric mass or a palpable gallbladder (Courvoisier's sign). The diagnosis is usually made with CT, MRI, endoscopic ultrasound, or endoscopic retrograde cholangiopancreatography (ERCP). Surgery is an option in a small percentage of cases. The Whipple procedure involves removing the head of the pancreas and part of the small intestine. The procedure is complicated and high-risk. The prognosis for pancreatic cancer is poor.

Hematology/Oncology

Anemia

Iron deficiency anemia

Iron deficiency anemia is one of the most common forms of anemia. It is especially common in women and pregnant women. Causes include blood loss (menstrual bleeding, GI bleed), a diet deficient in iron, difficulty absorbing iron (Crohn's disease, celiac disease), and increased demand (pregnancy). Patients are often asymptomatic if the anemia is mild. More severe anemia presents with fatigue, pallor, weakness, and headaches. Severe anemia causes pica, inflammation, and soreness of the tongue, cracks and fissures at the corners of the mouth, and poor appetite. The diagnosis is made by laboratory studies showing hemoglobin less than 10 g/dL for women and 12 g/dL for men. The peripheral blood smear will show a microcytic, hypochromic anemia. Serum ferritin and iron are low and the reticulocyte count is elevated. Treatment involves detecting and treating the underlying cause and oral iron replacement therapy.

Sideroblastic anemia, anemia of chronic disease, and hemolytic anemia

Sideroblastic anemia is caused by a failure to completely synthesize heme molecules, leading to deficient production of red blood cells. Causes include genetic abnormalities, drugs (alcohol, isoniazid, chloramphenicol), vitamin B_6 deficiency, and lead poisoning. The diagnosis is made by the presence of ringed sideroblasts and basophilic stippling of peripheral smear. Serum iron and ferritin levels are increased. Treatment depends on the underlying cause. Transfusion is sometimes needed for severe anemia. Anemia of chronic disease is caused by a depressed bone marrow and decreased red blood cell production. It is generally a normocytic anemia. Ferritin is generally elevated and iron and total iron binding capacity (TIBC) are low. The underlying chronic disease should be treated, if possible. Erythropoietin is sometimes used. Hemolytic anemia is characterized by increased destruction of red blood cells. It can be intravascular or extravascular. There are genetic causes and numerous acquired causes. Laboratory exam may show schistocytes or spherocytes on peripheral smear, elevated reticulocyte count, and positive Coombs' test. Bilirubin may be elevated and jaundice may be present. Treatment depends on the cause.

Vitamin B_{12} deficiency and folate deficiency

Vitamin B_{12} deficiency and folate deficiency cause a macrocytic megaloblastic anemia. Vitamin B_{12} deficiency can result from inadequate intake or decreased absorption of Vitamin B_{12}. Pernicious anemia is the most common etiology. It is caused by antibodies directed against intrinsic factor, a protein necessary for Vitamin B_{12} absorption. Other causes are dietary deficiency (vegans) and presence of a tapeworm. Vitamin B_{12} deficiency can lead to neurologic symptoms, including peripheral neuropathy, ataxia, and dementia. The diagnosis is made by the presence of decreased Vitamin B_{12} levels and a positive Schilling test (anti-intrinsic factor antibodies). Treatment is Vitamin B_{12} supplementation, either orally or via IM injection. Folate deficiency can be caused by insufficient dietary intake, alcoholism, malabsorption (celiac disease, IBD), and increased demand (e.g., pregnancy). Certain medications, such as methotrexate and phenytoin, can also cause folate deficiency. The diagnosis is made by the presence of decreased folate levels. Treatment is with oral folate supplementation.

Review Video: Pernicious Anemia
Visit mometrix.com/academy and enter code: 353419

Sickle cell disease

Sickle cell disease is an autosomal recessive disorder in which there is a mutation in the gene coding for the ß-chain of hemoglobin. A patient who is homozygous for the mutation has sickle cell disease. If they have only one copy of the mutation, they have sickle trait. The disease is most often seen in black people and Hispanics. The disorder results in sickling of red blood cells, which cannot flow as readily through blood vessels. This causes obstruction and deprives tissue of oxygen. Most patients are diagnosed by age 2 years. They present with anemia, acute pain crisis, stroke, acute chest syndrome, and splenic sequestration. Infections are frequent, especially pneumonia, which may be life threatening. The diagnosis is made by hemoglobin electrophoreses. Peripheral smear may show Howell-Jolly bodies, sickle cells, and target cells.

Management

Sickle cell disease is a lifelong illness that requires close management by a physician. Bone marrow transplant may cure it; however, most patients do not have a suitable donor and the risks are high. Treatment goals are to minimize complications and treat an acute crisis. Patients should receive both conjugate and polysaccharide pneumococcal vaccines and prophylactic penicillin. Hydroxyurea can be used to decrease the frequency of pain crisis. Acute crisis is managed with hydration, oxygen, and pain management. Transfusions are frequently necessary. Life expectancy is decreased. Most patients live to the fifth decade.

Review Video: Sickle Cell Disease
Visit mometrix.com/academy and enter code: 603869

Thalassemia

The thalassemias are a group of autosomal recessive inherited blood disorders that result in inadequate production of either the alpha- or beta-chain of hemoglobin. The alpha thalassemias are more common in individuals from Southeast Asia and China. There are four genetic loci that code for the alpha chain and the condition varies depending on how many loci are affected. If all four are affected, the condition is lethal in utero. If three are affected, hemoglobin H disease results, which leads to a moderate to severe anemia. If two loci are affected, the patient is said to have thalassemia minor. These patients have a mild anemia and normal life expectancy. If only one locus is affected, the patient is a silent carrier. Beta-thalassemia is most often seen in people of Mediterranean decent. There are only two beta hemoglobin alleles. If both are affected, the patient has beta-thalassemia major or Cooley's anemia. This is a severe anemia and leads to a shortened life expectancy. If one allele is affected, the patient has beta-thalassemia minor or trait. This causes a mild, asymptomatic anemia. Thalassemia carriers have some protection against malaria.

Thrombotic thrombocytopenic purpura

Thrombotic thrombocytopenic purpura (TTP) is a rare disease characterized by microthrombi, decreased circulating platelets leading to prolonged bleeding, and purpuric skin lesions. It can be inherited or acquired. The inherited form of the disease is caused by an abnormality in the gene that codes for the enzyme ADAMTS13. The acquired form is associated with pregnancy, HIV, certain cancers, and autoimmune disorders. Patients present with a hemolytic anemia, purpuric skin lesions, neurologic abnormalities and sometimes, renal disease. Treatment is with corticosteroids, plasmapheresis, and splenectomy. The prognosis is good for the first episode of the disease. If TTP recurs, the prognosis is poor.

Idiopathic thrombocytopenic purpura

Idiopathic thrombocytopenic purpura is an autoimmune platelet disorder that typically affects children and young adults. It can be acute or chronic. Patients present with bleeding, petechiae, and purpura. Treatment is with steroids, IVIG, and occasionally splenectomy. The prognosis is good.

Von Willebrand's disease

Von Willebrand's disease is the most common inherited clotting disorder. It is caused by a deficiency of von Willebrand's factor. It is an autosomal dominant disease that affects approximately 1% of the population. Men and women are equally affected. Patients may be asymptomatic or have mild symptoms such as prolonged nosebleeds, increased menstrual bleeding, or excessive bleeding following a cut or surgical procedure. There are three types of von Willebrand's disease (type 1, 2 and 3) characterized by decreasing to absent levels of von Willebrand's factor and increasing severity of symptoms. Patients generally have an increased bleeding time, increased PTT, decreased von Willebrand's antigen and decreased factor VIII activity. Treatment is DDAVP, von Willebrand's factor replacement, or factor VIII concentrate. Antifibrinolytics may be used for surgical procedures.

Disseminated intravascular coagulation

Disseminated intravascular coagulation (DIC) is also known as consumptive coagulopathy. Disseminated intravascular coagulation is characterized by simultaneous massive thrombosis and hemorrhage. It is generally seen as a complication in patients who are critically ill, such as in sepsis, trauma, malignancy, and certain obstetrical complications. Patients can present with petechiae and oozing of blood from wounds or with massive bleeding. Patients can also present with signs of thrombosis, including deep vein thrombosis (DVTs), digit ischemia, and necrosis. End organ damage may result, including liver and kidney failure. Laboratory work will show increased fibrin split products, D-dimer, and elevated PT/PTT. Fibrinogen, platelet count, hemoglobin, and hematocrit will all be low. Treatment should be aimed at correcting the underlying problem. Supportive measures include platelet transfusion, cryoprecipitate, and fresh frozen plasma (FFP).

Blood transfusions

Blood transfusion involves the transfer of blood or blood products from donor to recipient. Blood products used include: whole blood, packed RBCs, washed, irradiated or leukocyte-depleted RBCs, platelets, FFP, and cryoprecipitate. If a transfusion is anticipated, a type and cross should be performed. Transfusion carries risks of transmission of infections (CMV, HBV, HCV, and HIV) as well as transfusion reactions and should only be done when necessary. Directed donation by the patient, friends, or family members should be considered if the need for transfusion is anticipated well in advance.

The most common transfusion reaction is a febrile non-hemolytic reaction. Patients develop fever and chills during or shortly after a transfusion. Allergic reactions are also common. Delayed hemolytic reactions arise in about 0.1% and occur 2 to 5 days post-transfusion. Acute hemolytic reactions are rare and usually due to medical error. Patients present with fever, chills, hypotension, and possibly DIC within 24 hours. If a reaction occurs, the transfusion should be stopped immediately and the product sent back to the blood bank. A repeat type and cross should be performed.

Review Video: Blood Transfusions
Visit mometrix.com/academy and enter code: 759682

Polycythemia vera

Polycythemia vera is a disorder characterized by overproduction of red blood cells in the bone marrow. Most patients with polycythemia vera have a mutation in the gene encoding the protein JAK2. The disorder is usually seen in older adults. Initially, patients are often asymptomatic. As the disease progresses, patients develop headache, dizziness, itching, redness of the skin, and chest pain. Patients also can have splenomegaly, erythromelalgia, gout, and hypertension. Laboratory workup is significant for an increased hemoglobin and hematocrit, increased number of red blood cells, and low levels of erythropoietin. Bone marrow biopsy shows a hypercellular marrow with elevated numbers of megakaryocytes. Treatment options include serial phlebotomy, low-dose aspirin, hydroxyurea, and anagrelide. Complications include thrombosis, pulmonary embolism, stroke, and splenomegaly. Transformation to acute myelogenous leukemia occurs in 2% to 5% of patients.

Multiple myeloma

Multiple myeloma is a cancer of plasma cells. There is an increased risk in people over the age of 50 years, male, black people, and obese individuals. Patients diagnosed with monoclonal gammopathy of undetermined significance (MGUS) are at increased risk of developing multiple myeloma. Initially, patients are often asymptomatic. As the disease progresses, patients complain of bone pain, fatigue, loss of appetite, nausea, and weakness. The diagnosis is made by the presence of an M spike on serum protein electrophoresis. M proteins can also be found in the urine (Bence Jones proteins). Bone marrow examination is indicated. Asymptomatic patients do not require treatment. For symptomatic patients, treatment options include chemotherapy, corticosteroids, and stem cell transplantation. Complications include kidney failure, hyperviscosity syndrome, anemia, and immune deficiency. The median survival is 1 to 6 years.

Leukemia

Acute leukemia

Acute leukemias are rapidly progressive cancers of the blood or bone marrow. Presenting symptoms can include fatigue, easy bruising, bleeding, and frequent infection. The types of acute leukemia are:

- Acute lymphocytic leukemia (ALL), which is more common in children than adults with a peak between ages 2 to 5 years. Down's syndrome patients are at increased risk. Leukemic cells can be T-cells or B-cells. Treatment options include chemotherapy and bone marrow transplant. Long-term survival is 66% to 85% for children and 30% for adults.
- Acute myelogenous leukemia (AML), which is primarily a disease of adults over the age of 60 years. Smokers are at increased risk. Presenting symptoms may include leukostasis and blast crisis, and leukemia cutis (skin infiltration by leukemic cells). The presence of Auer rods in myeloblasts is diagnostic. Treatment options include chemotherapy and stem cell transplantation. The prognosis is poor with a five-year survival rate of 10% to 35%.

- Acute promyelocytic leukemia (APL), which is a subtype of AML. It primarily affects adults and is known for its sensitivity to all trans retinoic acid (ATRA), which produces remission in 90% of patients.

Chronic leukemia

Chronic lymphocytic leukemia (CLL) is a cancer of B-cells. It is the most common adult leukemia and typically affects people over the age of 50 years. Patients are often asymptomatic at diagnosis. The disease usually progresses slowly and treatment is not initiated until a patient is symptomatic. Symptoms can include fever, night sweats, weight loss, fatigue, lymphadenopathy, and hepatosplenomegaly. Treatment of symptomatic disease is with chemotherapy (generally with oral alkylating agents) or monoclonal antibodies. Chronic myelogenous leukemia (CML) is a rare cancer that affects primarily adults. Women are affected more often than men. It is associated with the Philadelphia chromosome t(9;22). Most patients are asymptomatic at diagnosis. The diagnosis is made by peripheral blood smear examination. Stage of disease is determined by the percentage of blast cells on peripheral smear. Treatment is initiated in the accelerated phase and includes imatinib mesylate (Gleevec®), stem cell transplant, and interferon-alpha. The median survival is 4 to 6 years.

Review Video: Leukemia
Visit mometrix.com/academy and enter code: 940024

Hodgkin's lymphoma

Hodgkin's lymphoma is less common than non-Hodgkin's lymphoma. It is characterized by the proliferation of Reed-Sternberg cells, a B-cell malignancy. Peak incidence is bimodal. It is seen in young adults (15 to 35 years) and again in adults over the age of 55 years. It is slightly more common in men. Risk factors include a positive family history and being immunocompromised. Most patients present with an enlarged, painless, lymph node. Other presenting symptoms include fever, night sweats, pruritus, and unexplained weight loss. The diagnosis is made by biopsy. Once diagnosed, the disease is staged. Treatment options include radiation, chemotherapy, and bone marrow transplant.

Non-Hodgkin's lymphoma

Non-Hodgkin's lymphoma is more common and a more aggressive disease than Hodgkin's lymphoma. It can occur at any age, but is more common in individuals over the age of 60 years. Acquired immune deficiency syndrome patients and people who are immunosuppressed are at increased risk. It can involve B-cells or T-cells. It is classified as indolent, aggressive, or highly aggressive. Aggressive and highly aggressive diseases have better cure rates than indolent disease. Presenting symptoms include a painless, enlarged lymph node, night sweats, unexplained weight loss, and pruritus. The diagnosis is made by biopsy. Burkitt's lymphoma is a form of non-Hodgkin's lymphoma. It is endemic in parts of Africa and usually related to Epstein-Barr Virus (EBV) infection.

Review Video: Lymphoma
Visit mometrix.com/academy and enter code: 513277

Primary brain tumors

The following are the most common primary brain tumors:

- Gliomas are tumors of glial cells and are the most common brain tumor. Ependymomas, astrocytomas, and oligodendrogliomas are all types of gliomas. They are also classified by grade, with glioblastoma multiforme being the most malignant. Presenting symptoms include headache or seizure. Treatment is generally a combination of surgery, chemotherapy, and radiation. Prognosis is generally poor.
- Medulloblastomas are highly malignant tumors of embryonal cells. They generally arrive in the cerebellum and are more common in children. Treatment is resection followed by chemotherapy. The five-year survival rate is about 80%.
- Meningiomas are usually benign, but can cause problems if they are large. They are most often seen in adults over the age of 60 years and are more common in women. Treatment is with surgical resection and it is often curative.

Bladder cancer

Painless hematuria in a patient over the age of 40 years is almost diagnostic for bladder cancer. Risk factors for bladder cancer include smoking, chronic cystitis, history of chemotherapy or radiation, and exposure to certain chemicals. Diagnosis is generally made by cystoscopy. Computerized tomography, intravenous pyelography (IVP), and ultrasound are also used. Treatment of superficial bladder cancer is with transurethral resection of the bladder tumor (TURBT) and intravesical BCG. Invasive bladder cancer is usually treated with radical cystectomy followed by chemotherapy.

Renal cell carcinoma

Renal cell carcinoma is the most common tumor of the kidney in adults. The classic triad of presenting symptoms is hematuria, flank pain, and an abdominal mass. Many patients are asymptomatic at diagnosis. Individuals with Hippel-Lindau syndrome are at increased risk. Treatment involves nephrectomy and immunotherapy with interferon-alpha or interleukin-2. Chemotherapeutic agents are not effective.

Cervical cancer

Women are recommended to begin cervical cancer screening with PAP smears three years after the onset of sexual intercourse, but not later than the age of 21 years. Women should continue to be screened annually until the age of 30 years and then every 2 to 3 years. After the age of 65 to 70 years, a woman may discontinue screening if she has had at least three consecutive negative PAP tests and no history of a positive test within the past ten years. Human papillomavirus (HPV) testing should be done, as HPV infection leads to an increased risk of cervical cancer. All abnormal PAP smears need to be followed up with either a repeat test or colposcopy, depending on the specific results. Treatment and prognosis depend on the stage of the disease at diagnosis.

Ovarian cancer

Ovarian cancer is the most deadly of the gynecologic cancers. Risk factors for developing ovarian cancer include a positive family history, not having children, and age over 70 years. Inheriting one of the breast cancer genes (BRCA1 or BRCA2) increases the risk. The use of hormone replacement therapy may increase the risk of ovarian cancer. The use of oral contraceptives lowers the risk. Patients are generally asymptomatic until the disease is advanced. Patients then present with abdominal swelling, bloating, and indigestion. The diagnosis is made by abdominal ultrasound and elevated CA-125 level. The treatment is surgery and chemotherapy. The prognosis depends on the stage of disease at diagnosis, but is often poor.

Infectious Disease

Bacterial meningitis

Meningitis is an inflammation of the meninges. The specific bacterial agent responsible for meningitis varies with different age groups. The most common pathogens in infants are Group B strep, *E coli,* and *Listeria*. *Neisseria meningitidis* and *Streptococcus pneumoniae* are the most common causes in children and young adults. Adults over the age of 50 years with meningitis most often have *S pneumoniae, Listeria monocytogenes*, and gram-negative bacilli. Presenting symptoms include high fever, severe headache, nuchal rigidity, and altered mental status. Patients may also complain of nausea, vomiting, and photophobia. On physical exam, findings include petechial or purpuric rash, neurologic deficits, Kernig's sign (pain is elicited with passive leg extension when thigh and knee are flexed), and Brudzinski's sign (passive flexion of the neck causes flexion of the hip and knee). Infants present atypically with irritability, poor feeding, and possibly a bulging fontanel.

Treatment and prognosis

Rapid diagnosis of bacterial meningitis is essential for effective treatment. The diagnosis is made based on the history, physical exam findings, CBC, and results of a lumbar puncture. Examination of the cerebral spinal fluid (CSF) typically shows a high protein and low glucose level. White blood cell count is usually $>300/mm^2$. Treatment is with IV antibiotics. Coverage should be broad until a specific organism is identified and sensitivity tests are available. A third generation cephalosporin sometimes combined with vancomycin (infants) or ampicillin (elderly) is used initially. Steroids are also sometimes used. Complications include shock, disseminated intravascular coagulation (DIC), abscess formation, and neurologic sequelae. The prognosis depends on length of time until diagnosis. A delay in diagnosis increases the chances of a bad outcome.

Viral meningitis

Viral meningitis refers to viral infection of the meninges. It is more common and usually milder than bacterial meningitis. Patients generally complain of severe headache, fever, nausea, and vomiting. Nuchal rigidity is less common than it is in bacterial meningitis. Numerous viruses can cause meningitis; however, enteroviruses are responsible for most cases. Enteroviral infection is most prevalent in the summer months. The diagnosis is made by lumbar puncture and CSF examination, which typically shows a normal glucose level and normal or slightly elevated protein. White blood cell count is usually $<300/mm^2$. Treatment is largely supportive care and most patients recover fully.

Conjunctivitis

Conjunctivitis is an inflammation of the conjunctiva. Causes include infection (both viral and bacterial), allergies, chemicals, and foreign bodies. Infectious causes predominate with viral causes being the most common. Patients present with conjunctival erythema, discharge, and photophobia. Distinction between viral and bacterial etiologies can be difficult. Viral cases are more commonly bilateral and show a clear watery discharge. Patients often have symptoms of an upper respiratory infection. Bacterial infections usually cause a unilateral purulent discharge. Culture of the discharge is sometimes indicated. Treatment of viral conjunctivitis is with cool compresses; bacterial cases require topical antibiotics. The most common pathogens include *Streptococcus, Staphylococcus*, and *Haemophilus influenzae*. Topical erythromycin, polymyxin, and trimethoprim preparations are frequently used.

Orbital and periorbital cellulitis

Periorbital (or preseptal) cellulitis is inflammation of the eyelid and skin surrounding the eye. Orbital cellulitis is inflammation of the orbit. Presenting symptoms of periorbital cellulitis include erythema and swelling of the eyelid and skin surrounding the eye. Orbital cellulitis presents with erythema, swelling, fever, and proptosis. Patients with orbital cellulitis often have pain, restricted extraocular movement, and decreased visual acuity. It is critical to differentiate between periorbital and orbital cellulitis. If orbital cellulitis is a possibility, CT scan, CBC, and blood cultures may aid in making the diagnosis. Periorbital cellulitis can be treated with oral antibiotics. Orbital cellulitis requires hospital admission and IV antibiotics. Antibiotic treatment should be broad-spectrum and cover staph and strep. Complications of orbital cellulitis include CNS infection and cavernous sinus thrombosis.

Sinusitis

Sinusitis is the inflammation of the sinus cavities. Sinusitis can be acute or chronic. Chronic sinusitis involves symptoms lasting longer than four weeks. Sinusitis can be viral or bacterial. The majority of cases (80%) are viral. The most common causes of acute bacterial sinusitis include *S pneumoniae*, *H influenzae*, *S aureus*, and *Moraxella catarrhalis*. Chronic sinusitis can be caused by anaerobes and *Pseudomonas*. Presenting symptoms include facial pain, fever, cough, and purulent nasal discharge. It can be difficult to distinguish viral from bacterial sinusitis. When symptoms persist for more than two weeks, the cause is usually bacterial. The diagnosis is generally based on the history and physical exam. In resistant cases, a CT scan is sometimes indicated. Treatment includes decongestants and antibiotics. Oral amoxicillin or Augmentin® are frequently used. Acute bacterial sinusitis requires 10 days of therapy; chronic sinusitis can require 3 to 4 weeks of oral antibiotics.

Acute pharyngitis

Acute pharyngitis is due to the inflammation or infection of the pharynx and/or tonsils. Most cases of pharyngitis are viral, and the second most common cause is bacterial. Other causes include allergies, gastroesophageal reflux and, rarely, tumors. Typical presentation of viral pharyngitis includes throat pain, low-grade fever, cough, and nasal discharge. Bacterial pharyngitis presents with fever >38°C, severe throat pain, headache, nausea, and vomiting. A purulent exudate is often present upon examination of the pharynx. The most common cause of bacterial pharyngitis is *S pyogenes* (group A streptococcus). Diagnosis is made by rapid antigen testing. Culture is indicated if the rapid test is negative. The treatment of choice is penicillin. Erythromycin is used in penicillin-allergic patients. Acute mononucleosis must be considered in the differential diagnosis.

Bronchitis

Bronchitis is an inflammatory condition of the trachea and bronchi. Acute bronchitis is most often caused by a virus. The most common viral causes include RSV, rhinovirus, adenovirus, and influenza. Bronchitis can also be caused by atypical bacteria, such as *Mycobacterium pneumoniae* and pertussis. Patients usually present with a history of cough, sometimes productive of sputum. Chest exam findings vary from clear to diffuse wheezes and rhonchi. Chronic bronchitis is usually related to smoking. Diagnosis is usually made clinically. Occasionally a chest x-ray is needed to rule out a focal pneumonia. Treatment of viral bronchitis is supportive care. Antibiotics should be used only if there is strong evidence to suspect a bacterial cause, or if the patient is elderly, compromised or a smoker.

Influenza

Influenza is a respiratory infection caused by influenza A or influenza B virus. Influenza epidemics typically occur in the winter. Influenza virus is also responsible for pandemics. Very young, elderly, and people with chronic illness are particularly susceptible to severe infection. The virus is spread via respiratory droplets and the transmission rate is high. Typical symptoms of the flu include fever, chills, headache, cough, weakness, and myalgias. The diagnosis is usually made clinically. Viral testing, either rapid antigen testing or culture, can be used to confirm the diagnosis. Treatment is generally supportive. Antiviral therapy should be started within the first forty-eight hours of illness. Prevention with annual vaccination of high-risk patients is important for minimizing morbidity and mortality.

Community-acquired pneumonia

Community-acquired pneumonia is pneumonia that develops in an individual who does not have a recent history of hospitalization. Patients typically present with fever, shortness of breath, and a productive cough. The workup should include a chest x-ray, CBC, blood cultures, and sputum for gram stain and culture. The most common organisms responsible for community-acquired pneumonias are:

- Streptococcus pneumoniae – most common organism
- *Haemophilus influenzae* – second most common cause
- *Staphylococcus aureus* – causes about 5% of community-acquired pneumonias
- *Legionella*
- Gram-negative rods – aspiration pneumonias
- *Mycoplasma pneumoniae*
- *Chlamydia pneumoniae*

Treatment is appropriate antibiotic therapy and supportive care. Patients with significant respiratory distress, hypoxemia, signs of shock, or inability to keep down oral fluids and medications require hospitalization and IV therapy. Complications include septicemia, pleural effusions, and lung abscess.

Hospital-acquired pneumonia

Hospital-acquired pneumonia is a pneumonia that develops in a patient that is either currently hospitalized or recently discharged. It is also known as nosocomial pneumonia. The pneumonia must develop at greater than forty-eight hours post-admission to be considered hospital-acquired. The most common organisms in hospital-acquired pneumonia are *S aureus*, *Pseudomonas*, *Enterobacter*, *Klebsiella*, and *Acinetobacter*. Patients usually present with fever, productive cough, and respiratory distress. Patients can sometimes present with mental status changes. The diagnosis is made by chest x-ray and blood and sputum culture. If the patient is on a ventilator, an endotracheal aspirate should be obtained. Treatment is with IV antibiotics and should be based on culture results. The mortality rate is 40% to 70%.

Hepatitis infections

Hepatitis A virus

Hepatitis A is typically less severe than other hepatitis infections. The virus is transmitted via the oral-fecal route and is frequently caused by contaminated food. Symptoms include fatigue, nausea, and vomiting, loss of appetite, RUQ abdominal pain, and jaundice. The diagnosis is made serologically. Acute infection will show an elevated IgM antibody. IgG will be elevated in patients with prior infection. Liver function tests should also be checked. Treatment is supportive care. Hepatitis A vaccination should be given to individuals who are traveling to high-risk locations, food handlers, day care workers, and patients with liver disease. Intravenous immunoglobulin (IVIG) should be given to close contacts of confirmed cases.

Hepatitis B

Hepatitis B affects millions of people worldwide. It is a serious disease leading to chronic infection in 5% to 10% of infected individuals. Fifteen to twenty percent of patients with chronic HBV will develop cirrhosis and liver failure, or hepatocellular carcinoma. The primary modes of transmission are sexual contact, needle sharing, and from an infected mother to her newborn. Patients with acute HBV infection present with flu-like symptoms, RUQ pain, and jaundice. Patients with chronic HBV may be asymptomatic. They may also show signs of cirrhosis and liver failure including ascites, jaundice, and spider angiomas. The diagnosis is made using serologic tests. The presence of an elevated anti-HBc IgG indicates past infection; anti-HBc IgM indicates acute infection. Hepatitis B surface antigen (HbsAg) is elevated in both acute and chronic infection. The level of hepatitis B envelope antigen (HbeAg) indicates viral load in the patient.

Treatment and prophylaxis: Treatment options include post-exposure prophylaxis with hepatitis B immunoglobulin (HBIG) along with the first dose of the vaccine. This should be given within 24 hours of exposure if possible. Infants born to hepatitis B positive mothers should receive HBIG in the delivery room and the first dose of the vaccine within 24 hours post-delivery. Treatment of patients with chronic HBV infection includes interferon, antivirals, and liver transplantation. Hepatitis B vaccine is now routinely given to all infants. The three-dose series is given post-birth, at the one-month visit, and at nine months. The vaccine should be given to all unimmunized older children and adults.

Hepatitis C

Hepatitis C virus (HCV) leads to chronic infection in approximately 75% of patients, 20% of which will go on to develop cirrhosis and liver failure. It is almost exclusively transmitted by infected blood and before the availability of screening assays, it was the most common cause of post-transfusion hepatitis. Acute infection is generally asymptomatic. Patients with chronic infection may have signs of liver failure. Diagnosis is made by the presence of HCV antibody. This will be detectable four to six weeks post-infection. Liver biopsy may be indicated to determine extent of disease and an appropriate treatment plan. Treatment consists of weekly subcutaneous pegylated interferon and twice daily oral ribavirin. Duration of treatment depends on genotype and ranges from 24 to 48 weeks. Liver transplant may be indicated in patients with severe end-stage liver disease. There is currently no HCV vaccine.

Infectious diarrhea

Most cases of infectious diarrhea are self-limited; however, globally it still remains community-acquired diarrhea should be assessed for signs of dehydration or presence of blood in the stool. Indications for further workup include dehydration, bloody stool, fever, an immunocompromised or elderly patient, and duration longer than one week. Stool should be sent for fecal leukocytes, culture, and O&P studies. Blood tests include CBC, electrolytes, and amoeba serology. Treatment of mild cases without significant dehydration includes oral rehydration and a diet that consists of bananas, rice, apples (juice or sauce), and toast (BRAT diet). Antidiarrheal agents are generally not indicated and may prolong the infection.

Antibiotic treatment

Antibiotic treatment of infectious diarrhea is indicated in the following cases:

- *Salmonella* – invasive disease, patients <3 months old, elderly, or immunocompromised. Use amoxicillin, trimethoprim/sulfamethoxazole (TMP/SZX), or cefotaxime.
- *Shigella* – all cases. Use TMP/SZX.
- *Yersinia* – cases with septicemia. Use TMP/SZX or ceftriaxone.
- *Campylobacter* – all cases. Use erythromycin.
- *E coli* – treatment not recommended for EHEC (0157) (enterohemorrhagic) and ETEC (enterotoxigenic). TMP/SZX is used for EPEC (enteropathogenic) and EIEC (enteroinvasive).
- *Giardia* – symptomatic disease should be treated with metronidazole or furazolidone.
- Amebiasis – all cases treated with metronidazole.
- AIDS related diarrhea – all cases must be treated.

Urinary tract infection

A urinary tract infection is an infection that occurs anywhere along the urinary tract. A lower urinary tract infection involving the bladder and urethra is known as cystitis. An upper urinary tract infection involves the ureters and kidneys. Classic presenting symptoms include urinary frequency, urgency, and dysuria. Hematuria and suprapubic pain may be present. Fever, flank pain, and tenderness are signs of upper urinary tract infection. Diagnosis is confirmed with urinalysis and culture. An uncomplicated UTI in an otherwise young, healthy non-pregnant female can be treated with a seven-day course of TMP/SMX or ciprofloxacin. A complicated UTI requires 10-14 days of treatment with a broad-spectrum antibiotic. Patients with upper UTI should be considered for hospitalization and IV antibiotics. Recurrent UTIs warrant further workup, including renal ultrasound and IVP.

Septic arthritis

Septic arthritis is an infection in the joint space. Risk factors for developing a septic arthritis include trauma, previous surgery, any type of immunocompromised state, and IV drug use. Patients typically present with fever, chills, and severe joint pain. There may be warmth, erythema, and decreased range of motion (ROM) of the infected joint. Workup should include CBC, blood culture, erythrocyte sedimentation rate (ESR), and C-reactive protein (CRP). Arthrocentesis should be performed and fluid sent for cell count, gram stain, and culture. Treatment includes drainage of fluid from the affected joint and appropriate IV antibiotics. A third generation cephalosporin should be used initially until results of culture and sensitivity are available.

Acute osteomyelitis

Osteomyelitis is an infection of the bone or bone marrow. Most cases of osteomyelitis result from trauma or surgery complications or in patients with vascular insufficiency, most commonly diabetes. Osteomyelitis can also result from hematogenous spread. Presenting symptoms include fever, pain, erythema, and swelling over the affected area. The workup should include CBC, blood cultures, ESR, and C-reactive protein. X-rays, bone scans, and MRI can be useful in making the diagnosis. Sometimes bone biopsy and culture are needed. The most common organisms depend on the specific situation of the patient. *Staphylococcus aureus* is the most common cause of osteomyelitis in patients who are post-op or have a prosthetic joint. Strep and anaerobes are seen following human bites and skin ulcers; *Pasteurella* is seen after an animal bite. *Salmonella* can cause osteomyelitis in sickle cell patients. Human immunodeficiency virus positive patients can develop *Mycobacterium*, *Bartonella*, or *Brucella* osteomyelitis. Treatment is 4 to 6 weeks of IV antibiotics, usually a third generation cephalosporin. Surgical drainage or debridement of necrotic tissue is sometimes indicated. Any foreign body should be removed, such as surgical plates or screws.

Splenectomized patient

Asplenic patients are at greater risk for overwhelming infection. A patient can be asplenic resulting from surgical removal of the spleen, or as the result of splenic dysfunction. The most common causes of functional asplenia are celiac disease, liver disease, and alcoholism. The presence of Howell-Jolly bodies on peripheral blood smear is strongly suggestive of functional asplenia. Postsplenectomy sepsis is an overwhelming, rapidly progressive condition that can quickly lead to shock and death. Patients that are either surgically or functionally asplenic should be vaccinated against pneumococcus, *H influenzae*, and meningococcus. Children and adolescents should receive penicillin prophylaxis for three years. Patients should be advised to report any fever to their physician.

Lyme disease

Lyme disease is one of the more common tick-borne illnesses. It is caused by the gram-negative spirochete *Borrelia burgdorferi*. The vector for transmission is the deer tick *Ixodes dammini*. It is most common in the Northeastern region of the US. Patients are often unaware of a tick bite. Presenting symptoms of Lyme disease include flu-like symptoms, migratory joint pains, and rash. The classic Lyme disease rash is known as erythema migrans. It generally appears as an expanding target lesion at the site of the tick bite. Approximately 70% to 80% of patients will exhibit the rash. The diagnosis can be difficult. Laboratory tests include the enzyme-linked immunosorbent assay (ELISA). The ELISA test has a high rate of false positive results so it must be confirmed with a western blot test. Polymerase chain reaction (PCR) testing is also available. Early stage disease is treated with a 14 to 21 day course of oral doxycycline, amoxicillin, or cefuroxime. Late-stage disease requires IV antibiotic treatment for 14 to 28 days. Complications include chronic joint pain and inflammation, Bell's palsy, peripheral neuropathy, and cardiac abnormalities including varying degrees of heart block.

Review Video: Lyme Disease
Visit mometrix.com/academy and enter code: 505529

Methicillin-resistant *S aureus*

Although previously an exclusively hospital-acquired infection, MRSA has become increasingly community-acquired. Methicillin-resistant *S aureus* is a strain of *Staphylococcus aureus* that is resistant to antibiotics. Overuse and inappropriate use of antibiotics may be responsible for the emergence of MRSA. Community-acquired infections are most likely spread from asymptomatic carriers. Patients generally present with pustular skin lesions, which can spread rapidly, leading to a life-threatening infection. The diagnosis is made by culture. The treatment depends on the sensitivity results of the patient's particular strain of MRSA. Vancomycin is frequently used.

Nephrology

Acute renal failure

Acute renal failure is a rapid loss of kidney function usually occurring over a period of days to weeks. Acute renal failure is generally accepted to be an increase in serum creatinine of 0.5 mg/dL, a 50% decrease in glomerular filtration rate (GFR), or the acute need for kidney replacement therapy. The causes can be grouped into three categories: prerenal, intrarenal, and postrenal. Prerenal causes include dehydration, hypotension, severe blood loss, shock, and sepsis. Heart failure and decreased cardiac output is also a cause. Intrarenal causes include renal artery or renal vein thrombosis, hemolytic uremic syndrome (HUS), glomerulonephritis, acute interstitial nephritis, and acute tubular necrosis (ATN). Toxins such as alcohol, cocaine, heavy metals, and certain chemotherapeutic agents can cause acute renal failure. Postrenal causes include urethral or bladder obstruction due to prostatic enlargement, stones, clots, or tumors.

Diagnosis and management

Presenting symptoms of acute renal failure includes decreased urine output, edema, shortness of breath, and seizures or coma in severe cases. The goal of the workup should be to make the diagnosis and identify the underlying cause. The workup should include a complete history and physical exam, including medication history as well as possible toxin exposure. The laboratory workup should include a U/A with microscopy, plasma electrolytes, BUN/creatinine, urine specific gravity, osmolality, and electrolytes. Renal ultrasound, CT or MRI are sometimes needed. Occasionally a renal biopsy will be needed to make the diagnosis. Treatment includes identifying and treating the underlying cause, giving adequate fluids, eliminating any nephrotoxic drugs, managing electrolyte abnormalities, and possibly administering dialysis.

Chronic renal failure

Chronic renal failure is abnormal kidney function of greater than three months duration or a glomerular filtration rate (GFR) of less than 60 mL/minute. The most common risk factor for developing chronic renal failure is diabetes. Other risk factors include hypertension, lupus, chronic glomerulonephritis, systemic lupus erythematosus, and sickle cell disease. Patients are often initially asymptomatic. Presenting symptoms are variable and nonspecific. They can include hypertension, decreased appetite, fatigue, weakness, edema, and decreased urine output. The diagnosis is based on laboratory tests, including tests measuring serum electrolytes, BUN/creatinine, U/A, and urine protein. Renal imaging studies and biopsy are also sometimes needed to make the diagnosis and determine the cause. Treatment involves treating the underlying condition and trying to halt progression. Angiotensin converting enzyme inhibitors (ACEIs) and angiotensin II receptor blockers (ARBs) are used to treat proteinuria and slow the progression of the disease. End-stage renal disease (GFR <15 mL/minute) is treated with dialysis or kidney transplantation.

Nephrotic syndrome

Nephrotic syndrome is a renal disorder in which the kidney allows a significant amount of protein to be lost in the urine. In nephrotic syndrome, there is no inflammation in the glomeruli. In general, proteinuria exceeding 3.5 grams per day per 1.73m^2 body surface area is considered a nephrotic syndrome. Nephrotic syndrome can be primary or secondary. Primary (idiopathic) causes include minimal change disease, focal segmental glomerulosclerosis (FSGN), membranous nephropathy, and membranoproliferative glomerulonephritis (MPGN). Secondary causes include diabetes, certain infections (HIV and HBV), malignancy, and amyloidosis. Presenting symptoms include loss of appetite, edema, frothy urine, and fatigue. The diagnosis is made by a 24-hour urine collection to quantify the level of proteinuria. Treatment includes angiotensin converting enzyme (ACE) inhibitors or angiotensin II receptor blockers (ARB) in order to reduce proteinuria. Edema is treated with diuretics. The underlying disease should be diagnosed and treated.

Nephritic syndrome

Nephritic syndrome is defined by the presence of hematuria, hypertension, signs of renal insufficiency, and edema. In nephritic syndrome, inflammation is present in the glomeruli. There are both primary (idiopathic) and secondary causes of nephritic syndrome. Primary causes include poststreptococcal glomerulonephritis (PSGN). This is the most common cause of nephritic syndrome. Other idiopathic causes include IgA nephropathy and anti-GBM disease. Secondary causes include systemic lupus erythematosus (SLE), Goodpasture's syndrome, and Wegner's granulomatosis. Patients often present with hematuria. Other presenting symptoms include anorexia, fatigue, and abdominal pain. Treatment is generally supportive care and the prognosis depends on the cause.

Hyponatremia

Hyponatremia involves having a plasma sodium of <135 mEq/L. Hyponatremia is usually secondary to some other disorder. Hyponatremia can be hypervolemic, euvolemic, or hypovolemic. This is determined by calculating the plasma osmolality and volume status of the patient. The plasma osmolality is calculated as follows: plasma osmolality = $(2\ [Na^+]) + ([BUN]/2.8) + ([glucose]/18)$. Causes of hyponatremia include kidney disease, excess free water intake, diuretics, SIADH, severe vomiting or diarrhea, low-sodium diet, liver disease, and congestive heart failure. Symptoms depend on the acuity and severity of hyponatremia. Patients may be asymptomatic. Symptoms can include nausea, vomiting, headache, and confusion. Severe cases can present with seizures and coma. Workup should include electrolytes, BUN, and glucose. Urine sodium should be determined. Treatment depends on volume status and underlying cause of the hyponatremia.

Hypernatremia

Hypernatremia involves having a serum sodium level >145 mEq/L. Hypernatremia can be caused by inadequate intake of water, such as with a defective thirst mechanism due to a hypothalamic problem or lack of access to water. It can also be caused by excessive water loss from sweating, GI losses, or burns. Hypernatremia can result from increased water losses from the kidney, as in diabetes insipidus. Patients may present with thirst or signs of dehydration. Other presenting symptoms include lethargy and weakness. In severe hypernatremia, patients may present with seizures or coma. The diagnosis is made based on the history, physical exam, and serum sodium level. Treatment is aimed at replacing the free water deficit. The free water deficit = total body water (TBW) x [(plasma Na/140) – 1]. The total body water is the patient's weight in kilograms multiplied by 0.6. Free water replacement can be accomplished orally in conscious patients who are able to drink or intravenously in more seriously ill patients.

Hyperkalemia

Hyperkalemia involves having an elevated serum potassium above the normal range (>5.0 mEq/L). Causes of hyperkalemia include excessive intake or excessive release from cells (e.g., trauma, burns, or tumor lysis syndrome). Hyperkalemia can also result from massive hemolysis. Insufficient elimination of potassium from renal insufficiency can also lead to hyperkalemia. Medications associated with hyperkalemia include ACE inhibitors, ARBs, potassium-sparing diuretics, NSAIDs, and heparin. Hyperkalemia is seen when there is a metabolic acidosis and in uncontrolled diabetes. Patients may be asymptomatic. Presenting symptoms can include weakness, muscle paralysis, and cardiac arrhythmias. Workup should include a serum potassium test and an EKG. Electrocardiogram findings may include peaked T waves, flattened P waves, prolonged QRS complex, and ventricular fibrillation in severe cases. Treatment options include Kayexalate®, diuretics, glucose and insulin, IV calcium gluconate, and dialysis.

Hypokalemia

Hypokalemia involves having a low serum potassium level (<3.5 mEq/L). Hypokalemia can result from inadequate intake, metabolic alkalosis, excessive GI losses, and excess renal excretion. Patients are usually asymptomatic until the potassium is below 3.0 mEq/L. Patients may present with muscle weakness and cardiac arrhythmias. The diagnosis is made by the presence of low serum potassium. A 24-hour urine collection for potassium may help determine the cause. Electrocardiogram findings may include flattened T waves, U waves, ST depression, and a prolonged QT interval. Treatment is potassium replacement. Oral replacement is appropriate for mild hypokalemia. Severe hypokalemia should be treated by the IV route, preferably with a central line.

Metabolic acidosis

Acidosis is defined as a pH of less than 7.35. A metabolic acidosis may or may not have an anion gap. The anion gap (AG) is calculated as follows: $AG = (Na^+) - [(Cl^-) + (HCO_3)]$. The anion gap is normally between six and ten. An anion gap greater than ten is evidence for an anion gap metabolic acidosis. A non-anion gap metabolic acidosis occurs when there is a loss of bicarbonate ion that is balanced with an increase in chloride. This is also called a hyperchloremic metabolic acidosis. A metabolic acidosis is usually caused by ingestion of a substance that either is an acid or can be metabolized into an acid. Examples include methanol, aspirin, and ethanol glycol. Diabetic ketoacidosis is also an example of a metabolic acidosis. Presenting symptoms include tachypnea, nausea, vomiting, and depressed mental status. Treatment is aimed at correcting the underlying cause. Bicarbonate therapy is used for severe acidosis (pH <7.10).

Metabolic alkalosis

Metabolic alkalosis is caused by an elevation in bicarbonate ions, leading to increased pH. Causes of metabolic alkalosis include GI acid losses from vomiting or NG tube suctioning, renal losses (e.g., hyperaldosteronism) or use of diuretics, sweat loss in cystic fibrosis, hypokalemia, and hypochloremia. Presenting symptoms are variable and dependent on the underlying cause. Severe metabolic alkalosis can cause headache lethargy, tetany, and seizures due to increased binding of ionized calcium. Treatment is aimed at the underlying cause. Chloride-responsive metabolic alkalosis (urine chloride <10 mEq/L) can be treated with a normal saline infusion. Chloride-unresponsive metabolic alkalosis (urine chloride >10 mEq/L) does not benefit from normal saline infusion. Severe alkalosis can be treated with acetazolamide or hydrochloric acid IV via a central line. The patient must be monitored with frequent arterial blood gases (ABGs) and electrolytes.

Respiratory acidosis and alkalosis

Respiratory acidosis involves increased carbon dioxide resulting from decreased ventilation. Causes include depressed respiration secondary to drugs, stroke or CNS infection, airway obstruction, intrinsic lung disease, or neuromuscular disorders such as multiple sclerosis or Guillain-Barré. A respiratory alkalosis is caused by decreased carbon dioxide levels because of increased ventilation. This can occur with CNS lesions, salicylate overdose, anxiety, and pain. Both respiratory acidosis and alkalosis are diagnosed using an arterial blood gas. Treatment is aimed at correcting the underlying cause.

Nephrolithiasis

Nephrolithiasis is the process of forming stones in the kidney or lower urinary tract. Risk factors for developing kidney stones include dehydration, family history, obesity, and hypertension. Kidney stones are more common in men. Patients generally present with bouts of severe back and flank pain, nausea, vomiting, dysuria, and hematuria. The diagnosis is made by helical CT scan. Workup should also include urinalysis, electrolytes, and urine for pH, calcium, oxalate, phosphorus, citrate, uric acid, and cysteine. Treatment includes increasing intake of fluids either orally or IV and observation to see if the stone passes spontaneously. Patients should be advised to strain their urine in order to identify the stone. If the stone does not pass, other treatment options include extracorporeal shock wave lithotripsy (ESWL), percutaneous nephrolithotomy, or removal via an ureteroscopic. Complications include urinary tract infection and renal damage.

Neurology

Headaches

Migraine headache

Migraine headaches are classified as either common migraines or classic migraines. The definition of common migraines is a syndrome of recurrent headaches that last from 4 to 72 hours and have at least two of the following qualities: unilateral, pulsatile, moderate to severe pain, aggravated by physical activity. There must also be nausea and/or vomiting or photophobia/hypersensitivity to sounds or smell. A classic migraine fulfills all of the above and is preceded by an aura. An aura is generally a focal neurologic event such as visual changes (bright light, flashing light, blind spots), auditory changes or focal numbness or tingling.

Management: Migraines are common, affect both men and women, and typically have their onset between the ages of 10 to 30 years. Patients present with a history of recurrent headaches with the above characteristics. The diagnosis is made by history and the presence of a normal neurologic exam. Computerized tomography, MRI, or lumbar puncture are occasionally needed to rule out other conditions. Depending on their frequency, migraines can be treated either acutely or prophylactically. Acute attacks can be treated with NSAIDs, triptans, ergotamines, narcotics, and antiemetics. Prophylactic medications include beta-blockers, calcium channel blockers, tricyclic antidepressants, and some anticonvulsant medications.

Tension headache

Tension headaches are the most common type of headache affecting most people at some point during their lifetime. Women are affected slightly more than men, and peak occurrence is between the ages of 20 to 50 years. Tension headaches are typically bilateral, have a band-like distribution, and are exacerbated by noise, fatigue, and stress. The diagnosis is made based on the history and a normal neurologic exam. Computerized tomography scan or MRI is occasionally indicated to rule out other causes of headache. Treatment of acute headaches is usually with acetaminophen or NSAIDs. Occasionally, severe tension headaches require narcotics. Frequent tension headaches can be treated prophylactically with antidepressants and beta-blockers.

Cluster headache

Cluster headaches are brief, but extremely painful, recurrent headaches that cause unilateral periorbital pain with conjunctival injection, tearing, runny nose, and ptosis of the affected eye. They are most common in middle-aged men. They sometimes occur in a cyclic manner at the same time every day. Acute treatments include 100% oxygen, triptans, ergotamine, intranasal lidocaine, and butorphanol. They can be treated prophylactically with prednisone, lithium, calcium channel blockers, and antidepressants.

Rebound headache

Rebound headache describes a pattern of daily headache associated with frequent use of pain medication. The headaches are bilateral, often associated with nausea, and occur daily, often in the morning. They are long in duration, frequently lasting the entire day. Treatment involves breaking the cycle of pain medication overuse.

Post-traumatic headache

Post-traumatic headaches are headaches that occur following minor head trauma. They present as generalized, constant, persistent headaches. Treatment is with analgesics and can be difficult to treat.

Temporal arteritis

Temporal arteritis, or giant cell arteritis, is a neurologic emergency. It is characterized by inflammation of the arteries of the head and neck. It most commonly occurs in women over the age of 50 years. Patients present with severe headache associated with visual loss or double vision, jaw pain, neck pain and stiffness, and sometimes fever and weight loss. On physical exam there may be dilated and tender temporal arteries. The diagnosis is usually made based on history and physical exam. Definitive diagnosis can be made by temporal artery biopsy. Erythrocyte sedimentation rate (ESR) is usually significantly elevated. Treatment is with prednisone, taken daily for 1 to 2 months. Complications include permanent visual loss, stroke, aortic aneurysm, and chest pain due to coronary artery inflammation. Aspirin can be used to reduce the risk of visual loss and stroke.

Pseudotumor cerebri

Pseudotumor cerebri (benign intracranial hypertension) is defined by presence of the triad of symptoms: headache, increased intracranial pressure (ICP), and papilledema in the absence of an identifiable cause. The symptoms mimic those of a brain tumor; however, no tumor is present. It is more common in women aged 20 to 40 years. Obesity is associated with an increased risk of developing pseudotumor cerebri. Patients generally present with severe headache and visual abnormalities, such as loss of vision, blurred vision, or double vision. Patients will sometimes have a depressed level of consciousness. The diagnosis is made by the presence of papilledema on physical exam and a CT or MRI which rules out the presence of a brain tumor. The scan may show slit-like ventricles. A lumbar puncture is significant for an elevated opening pressure. Treatment is with acetazolamide (Diamox®). Complications include permanent visual loss.

Intracranial arteriovenous malformation

Intracranial arteriovenous malformation is a congenital abnormality of the connections between the arterioles and venules in the brain. Patients are often asymptomatic and unaware they have an intracranial arteriovenous malformation until it bleeds. Patients occasionally will present with persistent headaches and seizures before the bleeding of an AVM. Hemorrhage of the AVM often leads to a change in mental status, signs of increased intracranial pressure, and focal neurologic symptoms. The diagnosis is made by MRI/MRA. Computerized tomography scan may show a hemorrhage. A lumbar puncture can be performed to look for evidence of a bleed. Treatment is with surgery or embolization if the AVM is not accessible. Mortality is about 10% if patients present with a bleed.

Stroke

Stroke is defined as the loss of brain function due to the interruption of blood supply to a particular region of the brain. Strokes can be thrombotic, embolic, or hemorrhagic. Strokes are very common. Risk factors include age >55 years, hypertension, hypercholesterolemia, smoking, diabetes, obesity, and having a family history or a personal history of stroke. Patients usually present with a sudden onset of a focal neurologic deficit. Presenting symptoms include difficulty with walking or speaking, focal weakness, paralysis or numbness, or visual problems. If stroke is suspected by history and physical exam, the diagnosis should be confirmed with a non-contrast CT or MRI.

Cerebral angiography can be performed to identify the site of the occlusion. Acute emergency treatment includes stabilization of the patient, anticoagulation with heparin or aspirin, and IV thrombolytic therapy with tissue plasminogen activator (tPA) in appropriate patients. The underlying cause of the stroke must be determined and treated.

Intracranial hemorrhage

Intracranial hemorrhage occurs when there is a disruption of an intracranial blood vessel. This can result from a ruptured aneurysm, trauma, or as a complication of anticoagulant therapy. Intracranial hemorrhage is a medical emergency. Presenting symptoms include sudden onset of a severe headache, nausea, vomiting, and mental status changes. Physical exam may show papilledema and focal neurologic deficits. The diagnosis can be confirmed with a CT scan. Treatment includes managing the increased intracranial pressure with hyperventilation, mannitol, and immediate neurosurgery.

Subarachnoid hemorrhage

Subarachnoid hemorrhage refers to bleeding into the subarachnoid space. The classic presentation is a patient who complains of "the worst headache of my life". Kernig's sign and Brudzinski's sign may be positive. The diagnosis can be confirmed by a CT scan. Treatment is with neurosurgery following stabilization of the patient.

Transient ischemic attack

Transient ischemic attack is defined as the sudden onset of a focal neurologic deficit that resolves within 24 hours. A deficit lasting 24 hours or longer is, by definition, a stroke. Transient ischemic attacks often last only a few minutes and leave no permanent deficits; however, they are considered warning signs of a potential stroke. Risk factors include hypertension, diabetes, hypercholesterolemia, smoking, advanced age, and family history. They are more common in men. Presenting symptoms are the sudden onset of a focal neurologic deficit, such as focal weakness or numbness, blindness in one eye, or speech problems. The diagnosis is made clinically. A CT scan is generally normal. A carotid ultrasound should be performed to evaluate the carotid arteries. Treatment options include anticoagulation and carotid endarterectomy.

Aphasias

Broca's aphasia, Wernicke's aphasia, and global aphasia

Aphasias are defined as the loss of the ability to produce or understand language, generally as the result of brain injury. Broca's aphasia is an expressive aphasia. Patients are unable to produce fluent, understandable language. Comprehension is intact. Wernicke's aphasia is a receptive aphasia. Patients are able to speak fluently; however, the content is often incorrect. Comprehension is poor. Global aphasia is a combination of both Broca's and Wernicke's aphasia, both language production and comprehension are impaired. It results from injury to both Broca's and Wernicke's areas of the cerebral lobe of the brain. The diagnosis of aphasias is made clinically. Treatment is with speech therapy and supportive care.

Focal seizures

Seizures result from abnormal activity of the brain. Focal seizures involve only part of the brain. Simple partial seizures do not cause the patient to lose consciousness. In complex partial seizures, there is a change in the level of consciousness. Focal seizures can be characterized by the region of the brain that is affected and the symptoms that are produced. Temporal lobe seizures are characterized by staring and unresponsiveness for several minutes. Patients usually experience an aura and a post-ictal period. Frontal lobe seizures typically last less than one minute and are characterized by unilateral clonic activity. Occipital lobe seizures are characterized by visual hallucinations. The diagnosis is based on the history and EEG findings. Treatment of acute seizures involves stabilization of the patient and IV benzodiazepines. Chronic seizures are managed with anti-epileptic medication.

Generalized seizures

Generalized seizures affect the whole brain and most cause a loss of consciousness. There are four types of generalized seizures: tonic clonic (grand mal), absence (petit mal), myoclonic, and atonic. Tonic clonic seizures are the most common. They are characterized by a tonic period (generalized stiffening) followed by generalized rhythmic jerking of the extremities (clonic phase). Incontinence and tongue biting are common. Absence seizures are more common in children. They are characterized by staring spells lasting 10 to 30 seconds. They show a characteristic spike and wave pattern on EEG. Myoclonic seizures consist of rapid brief contractions or jerking of muscles. There is no loss of consciousness. Electroencephalogram shows generalized polyspike and wave pattern. Atonic seizures are also known as drop attacks. They are characterized by sudden loss of muscle tone. All patients with a history of a new seizure should be worked up for an underlying cause with CBC, metabolic profile, and a toxicology screen. Computerized tomography scan or MRI should be performed to rule out tumors or bleeds. An EEG is also indicated.

Status epilepticus

Status epilepticus is defined as continuous seizure activity for greater than thirty minutes. Status epilepticus is a medical emergency. Patients need to be stabilized and establishment of an airway is critical. Intravenous access needs to be established. Medications that can be used to manage status epilepticus include benzodiazepines, phenytoin (Dilantin®), and fosphenytoin. Pentobarbital can be used if other treatments failed. If patients do not have a known history of epilepsy, a workup needs to be performed to find the underlying cause of the seizure. This includes CBC, metabolic profile, glucose, toxicology screen, and imaging studies. Complications of status epilepticus include respiratory failure, permanent brain damage, rhabdomyolysis, hyperthermia, and death.

Huntington's disease

Huntington's disease (Huntington's chorea) is an autosomal dominant progressive neurodegenerative disease that generally has its onset between the ages of 35 to 50 years and is fatal within 10 to 20 years. The patient usually has a history of a parent with the disease. Early symptoms of Huntington's disease include personality changes and cognitive difficulties. As the disease progresses, patients develop balance problems, chorea, speech and swallowing problems, and dementia. Computerized tomography scan shows cerebral atrophy. Genetic testing is available. Treatment is supportive care.

Creutzfeldt-Jakob disease

Creutzfeldt-Jakob disease is one of the transmissible spongiform encephalopathies. It is a degenerative brain disorder that is transmitted by prions. Patients initially present with personality changes and then develop a rapidly progressive dementia. The diagnosis is made by EEG, MRI, and biopsy. There is no effective treatment and patients generally die within a few months of diagnosis.

Guillain-Barré syndrome

Guillain-Barré syndrome is an autoimmune disorder characterized by progressive ascending muscle weakness beginning in the lower extremities. Guillain-Barré syndrome is often triggered by an infection, frequently *Campylobacter*. It can also be triggered by Hodgkin's disease, mononucleosis, and HIV. Patients present with a history of weakness and tingling sensations in their lower extremities. As the disease progresses, patients may develop shortness of breath, difficulty with bowel and bladder control, and eventually facial weakness and difficulty swallowing. Physical exam is significant for the absence of deep tendon reflexes in the lower extremities. Cerebral spinal fluid shows and an elevated protein count and a normal cell count. Electromyogram (EMG) is significant for slowed conduction velocity. The disease typically peaks in 2 to 3 weeks, but can have a much more rapid course and progress to respiratory failure in hours. Treatment includes plasmapheresis and IVIG. The mortality rate is 5%.

Carpal tunnel syndrome

Carpal tunnel syndrome is a compression neuropathy caused by entrapment of the median nerve. Risk factors for developing carpal tunnel syndrome include occupations that require repetitive wrist and finger movement. Carpal tunnel syndrome is more common in women, has a hereditary component, and is more common in individuals with diabetes, rheumatoid arthritis, and obesity. Patients present with a history of pain, tingling, and numbness in the first, second, and third digits, the distribution of the median nerve. Tapping on the median nerve may reproduce symptoms (Tinel's sign). Electromyogram and nerve conduction studies can aid in making the diagnosis. Treatment options include splinting, NSAIDs, and steroids. Surgery is indicated if medical treatment fails.

Amyotrophic lateral sclerosis

Amyotrophic lateral sclerosis (Lou Gehrig's disease) is a progressive neurodegenerative disease that is generally fatal in 3 to 5 years. Amyotrophic lateral sclerosis causes degeneration of both upper and lower motor neurons. The cause is unknown and most cases are sporadic. Symptoms can be subtle at first. Patients may have weakness or clumsiness. Patients eventually develop difficulty speaking, swallowing, and breathing. The cause of death is usually respiratory failure. The diagnosis is made clinically based on the presence of both upper and lower motor neuron dysfunction. Electromyogram can be used to confirm the diagnosis. Riluzole is the only drug available for treating ALS and there is some evidence that it may slow the progression of the disease. Otherwise, treatment is supportive care with physical and occupational therapy, nutritional and psychosocial support.

Review Video: Amyotrophic Lateral Sclerosis (ALS)
Visit mometrix.com/academy and enter code: 178603

Multiple sclerosis

Multiple sclerosis is an autoimmune disease that causes demyelination in the central nervous system. Multiple sclerosis is more common in women and generally has its onset between the ages of 20 to 40 years. The cause of MS is unknown. Genetic factors may be involved. It is more common in people of Northern European descent and there is an increased risk in children of MS patients. Presenting symptoms are highly variable. They include focal weakness, numbness and paresthesias, sudden blurring or loss of vision in one eye, tremor, lack of coordination, and unsteady gait. Focal deficits may be seen on neurologic exam. Magnetic resonance imaging (MRI) may show lesions in the white matter and lumbar puncture may show oligoclonal bands. The course of disease is highly variable and characterized by periods of remission and flare-ups. Treatment options include beta interferon, glatiramer, and natalizumab. Steroids are used to treat flare-ups. Physical therapy and supportive care should be offered.

Friedreich's ataxia

Friedreich's ataxia is an autosomal recessive progressive spinocerebellar disorder. It is generally diagnosed in childhood. Patients generally present in childhood with difficulty walking. The disease progresses to involve the arms and trunk. Eventually speech is affected and scoliosis develops. Depressed knee and ankle tendon reflexes are seen on physical exam. Magnetic resonance imaging may show spinal cord and cerebellar atrophy. Echocardiogram may be significant for ventricular hypertrophy. There is no effective treatment for Friedreich's ataxia. Supportive care to treat symptoms should be offered. Patients generally die by the age of 35 years.

Involuntary movement disorders

Chorea

Chorea is an involuntary movement disorder characterized by rapid, irregular movements of the hands and feet. Movements are often "dance-like". Explosive and inappropriate speech is sometimes present. Symptoms do not occur during sleep.

Athetosis

Athetosis is an involuntary movement disorder characterized by slow, writhing movements, generally of the hands or feet. The movements can be brought on by emotional stress or during specific activities. There are no symptoms during sleep.

Tremor

A tremor is an involuntary movement disorder characterized by rhythmic or oscillatory movements. A postural tremor occurs when there is a sustained posture of an extremity, for example, an outstretched arm for example. An intention tremor occurs when a purposeful movement is being attempted, such as touching a finger to the tip of one's nose for example. A resting tremor is a tremor that occurs at rest. Parkinson's disease is characterized by resting tremors.

Horner's syndrome

Horner's syndrome is caused by sympathetic nerve damage. Patients present with miosis, mild ptosis, and anhidrosis all on the affected side. Horner's syndrome is always caused by an underlying disease. Causes include tumor, stroke, and carotid artery dissection. Treatment is directed at the underlying cause.

Bell's palsy

Bell's palsy is a syndrome that results from facial nerve paralysis. Most cases are idiopathic. Bell's palsy can also be associated with Lyme disease, HIV, herpes, or other infections. Pregnant women and diabetics have an increased incidence of Bell's palsy. Patients present with the sudden onset of weakness or paralysis on the affected side of the face. Patients may complain of facial pain, headache, or loss of taste. The diagnosis is made clinically and a workup is needed to rule out a possible underlying cause. Treatment options include corticosteroids and antivirals. Most patients recover completely.

Ophthalmology

Red eye

There are many causes of red eyes. They include conjunctivitis, corneal abrasion, foreign body, blepharitis, preseptal and orbital cellulitis among others. Evaluation should start with a detailed history. A careful thorough eye exam should be performed, including careful inspection of the lid and surrounding structure, pupil, extraocular muscles, and visual acuity. Fundi should be visualized with an ophthalmoscope. A slit lamp exam should be performed if available and intraocular pressure should be measured. Decreased visual acuity, pupillary abnormalities, and abnormal intraocular pressure are signs of a potentially serious condition and ophthalmologic referral may be indicated. Specific treatment will depend on the diagnosis.

Corneal abrasion

Corneal abrasions result from trauma to the corneal epithelium, generally as the result of trauma or a foreign body. Patients generally present with pain, tearing, injection, and mild edema. They often complain of a sensation that there is a foreign body in their eye. The diagnosis is made by history and physical exam. The eye should be stained with fluorescein and examined under a Wood's lamp. The eye should be carefully examined for the presence of a foreign body. Treatment includes topical antibiotics and systemic analgesics. Patching and topical analgesia are not recommended. Severe cases or presence of a foreign body should be referred to an ophthalmologist. Complications include erosions, corneal ulcers, and visual loss.

Angle-closure glaucoma

Acute angle-closure glaucoma, also known as narrow-angle glaucoma, is a condition characterized by a sudden and rapid increase in intraocular pressure. This occurs when the iris blocks the drainage of aqueous humor from the eye. If left untreated, it can cause optic nerve damage and permanent visual loss. Patients present with the sudden onset of eye pain, profuse tearing, headache, and blurred vision. Patients may also have nausea and vomiting. The diagnosis is made based on the history and physical exam as well as the presence of increased intraocular pressure and the detection of the obstruction using gonioscopy.

Treatment involves topical agents to constrict the pupil and iridotomy. Immediate ophthalmologic referral is indicated.

Review Video: Glaucoma and Cataracts
Visit mometrix.com/academy and enter code: 279024

Hyphema and orbital fractures

A hyphema is defined as bleeding in the anterior chamber of the eye. Hyphema is usually the result of trauma. Patients present with a complaint of decreased visual acuity. Layering of blood in the anterior chamber can sometimes be seen by the naked eye. Diagnosis is made using ophthalmoscopic or slit lamp exam. Treatment is with bedrest and elevating the head of the bed. Complications include glaucoma and visual loss. An orbital fracture occurs when any one of facial bones that make up the orbit is broken. The diagnosis is made by CT scan. Treatment is surgery.

Orthopedics

Stress fractures

Stress fractures are common overuse injuries seen in athletes. They are frequently seen in runners and are more common in women. The lower extremity is usually affected, especially the tibia, fibula and bones of the foot. Patients present with a history of pain that initially occurs only towards the end of the workout. As the fracture worsens, the pain is experienced for longer periods of time. The affected area may be swollen and tender to the touch. The diagnosis is generally made clinically; x-rays may show a periosteal reaction. Treatment includes rest, ice, and pain medication. Immobilization may be indicated for severe cases.

Medial tibial stress syndrome

Shin splints (Medial tibial stress syndrome) are a condition characterized by pain along the tibia resulting from stress to the bone and surrounding tissues. It is commonly seen in runners and jumpers. Patients present with pain and tenderness along the medial portion of the tibia. The diagnosis is made clinically. Treatment includes rest, ice, and pain medication.

Slater-Harris classification of fractures

The Slater-Harris classification of fractures is a method of classifying fractures in children that affect their growth plate. The classification helps determine the treatment and prognosis. The classification is as follows:

- Type I is through the physis. The growth plate is rarely disturbed and the prognosis is excellent.
- Type II is through the physis and metaphysis. These are the most common fractures. They carry a risk of growth disturbance.
- Type III is through the physis and epiphysis. These fractures involve the joint and orthopedic referral is indicated.
- Type IV fractures are through the metaphysis, physis, and epiphysis. These fractures can often cause chronic growth problems.
- Type V are crush injuries.
- Type VI are injuries to the perichondrium.

Rotator cuff injuries

The rotator cuff consists of the subscapularis, supraspinatus, infraspinatus, and teres minor muscles, as well as the tendons connecting them to the humerus and scapula. Rotator cuff injuries are common and usually the result from falling or repetitive arm motions such as throwing a ball. The injury can consist of tears, tendonitis, or bursitis. Patients present with pain, shoulder weakness and decreased range of shoulder motion of the shoulder. Patients often have difficulty with abduction and internal rotation. The diagnosis is made based on the history and physical exam findings. An MRI is often used to diagnose a tear. Treatment generally consists of rest, pain medication, and physical therapy. Significant tears often require surgical repair.

Adhesive capsulitis

Adhesive capsulitis, or frozen shoulder, is a condition characterized by pain, stiffness and limited range of motion, both active and passive, of the shoulder joint. The etiology is generally not known.

There is an increased incidence in people over the age of 40 years, diabetics, after those who have had periods of prolonged immobility, and patients with thyroid disease, cardiovascular disease, and Parkinson's disease. Patients present in three stages. The initial stage is the painful stage, which is characterized by pain and decreased range of motion. During the frozen stage, pain decreases and range of motion is severely limited. During the thawing stage, range of motion begins to increase. The diagnosis is made clinically. An MRI may be indicated to rule out other conditions. Treatment consists of pain medication, steroid injections, and physical therapy. Surgery is rarely necessary.

Little League elbow

Little League elbow is a condition characterized by elbow pain generally as the resulting from of repetitive throwing. It is frequently seen in young (prepubescent) baseball pitchers. The injury involved is medial epicondyle apophysitis. The diagnosis is made clinically. Treatment is rest, pain medication, and physical therapy. Surgery is occasionally needed if there is ulnar neuropathy or valgus instability.

Nursemaid's elbow

Nursemaid's elbow is a very common injury seen in children under the age of 5 years. Nursemaid's elbow, or subluxation of the radial head, is a dislocated elbow often caused by pulling a child up by their arm. The annular ligament is lax in young children and more prone to displacement. The child presents holding the affected arm slightly flexed and pronated. The child generally refuses to move the arm. The diagnosis is generally made clinically. An x-ray may be indicated to rule out a fracture if the diagnosis is not clear. Treatment involves reduction. While supporting the radial head, the forearm is quickly supinated and flexed in one motion. If successful, the child will start using the arm immediately.

Mallet finger

Mallet finger, or jammed finger, results when there is forced flexion of an extended distal interphalangeal (DIP) joint. The injury frequently occurs while playing basketball or baseball. The diagnosis is made clinically. An x-ray should be performed to rule out a fracture. Treatment is extension splinting.

Jersey finger

Jersey finger is an injury to the distal interphalangeal joint often seen when a football player grabs the jersey of another player, leading to forced extension of the DIP joint. This causes an avulsion injury of the flexor digitorum profundus tendon. It is most often seen in the ring finger. Treatment is surgical repair.

Boutonniere deformity

Boutonniere deformity describes the abnormal position of hyperflexion of the PIP joint with hyperextension of the DIP joint. It can be caused by trauma or inflammatory conditions such as rheumatoid arthritis. Treatment is extension splinting.

Scoliosis

Scoliosis is defined as an abnormal lateral curvature of the spine (>10°). The vast majority of scoliosis cases are idiopathic. Risk factors for developing scoliosis include certain neuromuscular disorders such as cerebral palsy and vertebral disease such as tumors or infections. Severe scoliosis is more common in girls. Scoliosis is generally diagnosed by screening during routine physical exams. Signs include uneven shoulders and/or hips and leaning to one side. The diagnosis is usually made by physical exam. Spine x-rays should be performed to measure the degree of curvature. Mild scoliosis, <20° curvature, requires no treatment, but should be monitored closely for progression. More severe scoliosis can be treated with bracing. Surgery with spinal fusion is sometimes needed for severe cases. Complications include chronic back pain. Severe scoliosis can cause cardiac and pulmonary problems.

Knee injuries

Meniscal tear

A meniscal tear, or "torn cartilage", occurs when there is an injury to either the medial or lateral meniscus in the knee. This can occur as a result of trauma or due to a degenerative process that occurs with aging. Patients present with pain and swelling of the knee. A joint effusion may be present. The diagnosis is made by MRI. Treatment is surgery.

Anterior cruciate ligament tear

The anterior cruciate ligament is an important stabilizer of the knee. An ACL tear is one of the most common orthopedic injuries seen in athletes. It often results from sudden excessive rotational stress on the knee. Patients present with sudden onset of severe knee pain. Physical exam shows a positive Lachman test. Treatment options include rest and physical therapy, or surgical repair.

Collateral ligament injury

Collateral ligament injury (medial or lateral) is usually the result of trauma to the lateral aspect of the knee. Patients present with pain. There is increased laxity of the knee on physical exam. Tears are graded I to III depending on severity. Treatment includes rest, pain medication, physical therapy, and bracing.

Osteochondritis dissecans

Osteochondritis dissecans is a disorder characterized by necrosis and ultimately separation of subchondral bone. It most commonly occurs on the medial femoral condyle and it is the most common cause of a loose body in the joint space in pediatric patients. It is usually due to repetitive stress to the bone. It typically presents in teenage athletes, who complain of the gradual onset of vague knee pain. Pain may worsen and swelling may develop following physical activity. The diagnosis is usually made by x-ray or MRI. Stable lesions may be managed conservatively by modifying activity. More advanced unstable lesions are managed with surgery.

Plantar fasciitis

Plantar fasciitis is an inflammatory condition of the plantar fascia. Risk factors for developing plantar fasciitis include participation in sports, having flat feet, obesity, and pregnancy. It is more common in middle-aged individuals. Patients present with heel pain that is typically worst when they first get up in the morning. The diagnosis is usually made clinically. An x-ray or MRI may be needed to rule out other conditions. Treatment options include activity modification, night splints, orthotics, and steroid injections. Occasionally, surgery is needed to detach the plantar fascia from the heel (plantar fasciotomy). Complications include back, hip and knee pain as well as gait problems.

Rheumatoid arthritis

Rheumatoid arthritis is an autoimmune, chronic inflammatory disease of the joints. Rheumatoid arthritis is more common in women and is typically diagnosed between the ages of 40 to 60 years. Patients present with joint pain and swelling. The PIP, MTP joints, wrists, knees, and ankles are usually affected first. The elbows, shoulders, hips, and neck are affected later in the disease. Patients may also complain of morning stiffness, fever, and weight loss. The diagnosis is made by the presence of inflammatory arthritis in multiple areas, a positive rheumatoid factor, and the presence of rheumatoid nodules. X-rays may show characteristic changes in the joints. Rheumatoid arthritis is a chronic disease characterized by exacerbations and remissions. There is no cure; treatment is aimed at preventing progression and minimizing symptoms. Treatment options include NSAIDs, steroids, disease-modifying antirheumatic drugs (DMARDs), and immunosuppressants. Surgical joint replacement is sometimes indicated.

Gout

Gout is a disorder characterized by the deposition of uric acid crystal deposits around a joint or in other parts of the body. Risk factors for developing gout include excessive alcohol use, hypertension, diabetes, hyperlipidemia, and a positive family history. Use of thiazide diuretics, low-dose aspirin, and anti-rejection medications also increase the risk. It is more common in men. Patients typically present with the acute onset of severe joint pain in the first MTP joint. Gout can present in other joints also. The affected joint appears red and swollen. The diagnosis is made based on the history and physical exam. Synovial fluid examination may show urate crystals. Serum uric acid is usually elevated. Treatment options include NSAIDs, colchicine, and steroids. Patients with gout are at increased risk for developing urate kidney stones.

Obstetrics/Gynecology

Preconception counseling

The goal of preconception care is to maximize the chances for a healthy pregnancy. The preconception assessment should include questions about the patient's medical history, diet, medications, possible exposure to toxins, substance abuse history, family history, and psychosocial history. Special attention should be given to the patient's reproductive history, including method of contraception, previous pregnancies, and any history of sexually transmitted diseases. A complete physical exam should be performed, including a pelvic exam. Laboratory tests should include CBC, blood type, rubella titer, hepatitis B antigen, rapid plasmin reagin (RPR), *Chlamydia*, and PAP test. Other lab tests that should be considered include HIV, *Varicella*, glucose, PPD, and toxoplasmosis titer. In some patients, genetic testing for a particular disease may be indicated. Patients should be counseled to stop any potentially harmful medications, refrain from alcohol and smoking, and to begin prenatal vitamins.

Diagnosis of pregnancy

Pregnancy should be suspected in any woman of childbearing age whose menstrual cycle is disrupted. Early symptoms of pregnancy include nausea, vomiting, fatigue, and breast enlargement and tenderness. Physical exam findings include a blue discoloration of the cervix (Chadwick's sign), softening of the cervix (Goodell's sign), softening of the uterus (Ladin's sign and Hegar's sign), darkening of the nipples, and uterine enlargement. The diagnosis can be confirmed with urine beta-HCG assay. Pelvic ultrasound can also be used to confirm pregnancy. Assessment of gestational age and due date can be assessed by calculations using the date of the last menstrual period or by assessing fetal size using ultrasound.

Prenatal care

First trimester

The initial prenatal visit should include a complete physical exam, including a pelvic exam. If not performed at a preconception evaluation, the following laboratory exams need to be obtained: CBC, blood type, rubella titer, hepatitis B antigen, RPR, *Chlamydia*, and PAP test. Other lab tests that should be considered include HIV, *Varicella*, glucose, PPD, and toxoplasmosis titer. In addition, a U/A and culture and a 1-hour glucose tolerance test should be performed. Patients should be counseled regarding what to expect during pregnancy, diet including foods that must be avoided (e.g., raw fish, unpasteurized dairy products, soft cheese, fish potentially high in mercury), appropriate weight gain, and drug, alcohol and smoking cessation. Genetic testing should be discussed. Patients should be started on prenatal vitamins if not already initiated at a preconception visit.

Second and third trimester

Visits are typically monthly until 28 weeks, bimonthly from 28 to 36 weeks, and then weekly until delivery. At each visit during the second and third trimesters of pregnancy, the following should be performed: fundal height measurement, blood pressure, auscultate for fetal heart rate, palpate and attempt to determine fetal position. The final visits in the third trimester should include a digital cervical exam for opening and effacement. Laboratory tests include urine dipstick for glucose and protein at each visit. At 15 to 18 weeks gestation, genetic screening should be offered. A 1-hour glucose tolerance test should be performed at 26 to 28 weeks and group B streptococcus testing should be performed at 36 weeks. Patients should be counseled regarding the onset of labor, when to call their physician, and anesthesia options in the delivery room.

Hyperemesis gravidarum

Hyperemesis gravidarum is defined as extreme, unrelenting vomiting that prohibits intake of adequate food and fluids, leading to weight loss and ketonuria. Hyperemesis gravidarum affects approximately 1 in 200 pregnancies and it usually starts by 10 weeks gestation. Patients present with persistent nausea and vomiting, weight loss of >5% of body weight, and signs of dehydration. Risk factors include a prior history of hyperemesis gravidarum, multiple pregnancy, first pregnancy, and molar pregnancy. The workup should include an ultrasound, electrolytes, CBD, LFTs, TFTs, and U/A. Once other causes are ruled out, the diagnosis can be made. Treatment may require hospital admission, IV fluids, NG feeds, or possibly total parenteral nutrition (TPN). Antiemetics can be used for severe cases. The condition usually resolves by the end of the first trimester.

First trimester vaginal bleeding

Bleeding during the first trimester of pregnancy is not uncommon. Physiologic bleeding is usually light and self-limited. Causes include implantation and cervical changes or trauma following pelvic exam or sexual intercourse. The patient should be reassured, and generally, no further workup is needed. First trimester bleeding can also be a sign of a spontaneous or threatened abortion. The bleeding is usually moderate to heavy and is accompanied by uterine cramping. The workup should include a pelvic exam, ultrasound to assess the well being of the fetus, and a CBC. If a spontaneous abortion is diagnosed, uterine evacuation may be indicated.

Ectopic pregnancy

An ectopic pregnancy occurs when the fertilized ovum implants outside of the uterus, usually in the fallopian tubes. Approximately 1% of pregnancies are ectopic. Risk factors for ectopic pregnancy include: a history of a prior ectopic pregnancy, current use of an intrauterine device (IUD), history of salpingitis or pelvic inflammatory disease, structural anomalies of fallopian tubes or uterus, and current use of fertility drugs. Patients generally present with pelvic pain, light bleeding, and cramping. A tubal pregnancy may be silent until it ruptures, at which time patients develop severe abdominal pain. The diagnosis is made by positive urine pregnancy test and ultrasound, which shows an empty uterus. Treatment of small, non-ruptured ectopic pregnancy is IM methotrexate. A ruptured ectopic pregnancy is treated with surgical removal.

Placenta previa, placental abruption, and vasa previa

Placenta previa, placental abruption, and vasa previa are all potential causes of third trimester bleeding. Placenta previa occurs when there is a low-lying placenta such that it either partially or fully covers the opening of the cervix. Risk factors include age >35 years, multiple pregnancy, smoking, and previous uterine surgery, including history of a C-section and smoking. Patients present with painless bleeding. The diagnosis is made by ultrasound. Management may include bed rest and emergency C-section if heavy bleeding occurs. C-section is generally performed at about 34 weeks. Placental abruption is the separation of the placenta from the uterus before delivery. Placental abruption is a surgical emergency and it can be partial or complete. Patients generally present with severe bleeding and abdominal pain. Vasa previa occurs when fetal blood vessels lie between the fetus and the opening of the cervix. Patients present with painless bleeding. C-section is indicated.

Intrauterine growth retardation

Intrauterine growth retardation refers to a fetus whose weight is below the tenth percentile. There are many potential causes of IUGR. Placental abnormalities, maternal chronic disease, smoking, drug or alcohol abuse, as well as genetic anomalies of the fetus can all cause IUGR. IUGR is generally diagnosed at a prenatal visit when fundal height is not what is expected for gestational age. The diagnosis should be confirmed by ultrasound. Treatment options depend on the underlying cause. A full workup is needed to determine the etiology cause of IUGR. This may include a detailed ultrasound, fetal karyotype, and screening for maternal infection. Treatment options depend on the underlying cause. Steroids are sometimes used to speed fetal lung development.

Gestational diabetes

Gestational diabetes is defined as glucose intolerance that occurs only during pregnancy. Gestational diabetes is very common, affecting up to 14% of pregnancies. Women at higher risk include those who are overweight, have a personal or family history of diabetes, and black, Hispanic, American Indian, and Asian women. Affected women are generally asymptomatic. Gestational diabetes is usually identified during routine screening. Gestational diabetes increases the risk of macrosomia, hypoglycemia, respiratory distress, jaundice, and subsequent development of type 2 diabetes in the fetus. Gestational diabetes also increases the risk of preeclampsia and polyhydramnios. Treatment options include dietary management and insulin if dietary measures do not control blood sugars. Close monitoring of blood glucose levels is essential.

Macrosomia, polyhydramnios, and oligohydramnios

Macrosomia is defined as a fetus weighing more than 4.5 kg. Maternal diabetes is the most common etiology. Common delivery complications include shoulder dystocia and maternal trauma. Polyhydramnios is defined as having excess amniotic fluid. Maternal diabetes is the most common cause. The risk of preterm labor is increased with polyhydramnios. Amniotic fluid reduction is sometimes indicated. Oligohydramnios is defined as having insufficient amniotic fluid. Maternal hypertension and diabetes are causes. It is often idiopathic. Diagnosis can be made by ultrasound. Management includes close monitoring, maternal hydration, and possibly amnioinfusion.

Premature rupture of membranes

Premature rupture of membranes is defined rupture of membranes before the onset of labor. This can occur at term or preterm (prior to 37 weeks gestation). Premature rupture of membranes is very common, affecting almost 10% of pregnancies. Risk factors include sexually transmitted diseases (STDs), smoking, and multiple gestations. Patients present with a history of clear fluid leakage from the vagina. Labor often begins within 24 hours of membrane rupture. The diagnosis is confirmed by checking the pH of the fluid (nitrazine testing), or looking for characteristic ferning of amniotic fluid under the microscope. Complications of PPROM include preterm delivery and infection. Treatment depends on gestational age and overall health status of the mother and fetus. Treatment options include hospitalization, tocolytics, antibiotics, and an expedient delivery if needed.

Preterm labor

Preterm labor is defined as the onset of contractions and cervical changes before 37 weeks gestation. Preterm labor and births are common, affecting approximately 10% of pregnancies. Risk factors include lack of prenatal care, smoking, drug or alcohol abuse, multiple gestation, uterine or placental abnormalities, maternal infection, and congenital anomalies of the fetus. Workup should include the measurement of fetal fibronectin in vaginal secretions. A positive result is indicative of fetal membrane detachment and impending preterm delivery. Management options for preterm labor include bed rest, corticosteroids to hasten lung maturity, and tocolytics. If maternal infection is present, appropriate antibiotics should be administered.

Preeclampsia

Preeclampsia, which is also known as pregnancy induced hypertension, is defined as the presence of hypertension and proteinuria after 20 weeks gestation. Risk factors for developing preeclampsia include a prior history, first pregnancy, age >35 years, obesity, multiple gestation, diabetes, kidney disease, or lupus. Patients may present with headaches, nausea, vomiting, dizziness, or decreased urine output. Physical exam may reveal peripheral edema. Blood pressure is >140/90 mm Hg and urine dips are positive for protein. A 24-hour urine protein test for protein should be obtained in patients whose dipstick is positive. The only cure for preeclampsia is delivery. If too early for delivery, management options for delivery include bed rest, antihypertensives, and $MgSO_4$. Complications include placental abruption, fetal demise, progression to eclampsia (preeclampsia with grand-mal seizures), and Hemolysis, Elevated Liver enzymes and Low Platelets (HELLP) syndrome.

Labor and delivery

Labor is defined as a process of increasingly frequent and intense uterine contraction leading to cervical effacement and dilation and ultimate delivery of the fetus and placenta. Normal labor is divided into three stages. Stage I begins with the onset of regular uterine contractions and ends when the cervix is fully dilated. Stage I is divided into a latent phase, an active phase, and transition. The latent phase is characterized by cervical dilation up to 3 cm, loss of the mucous plug, and contractions that are less intense and farther apart. The latent phase can last 14 to 20 hours. During the active phase, the cervix dilates to the range of 3 to 9 cm. Contractions are closer together and more intense. In transition, the cervix dilates to the range of 9 to 10 cm. Stage II involves descent and delivery of the fetus. Frequent exams to determine station and position of the fetus are critical. During stage III of labor, the placenta is delivered.

<u>Pain management</u>
There are several nonpharmacologic methods for controlling labor pain. They include relaxation techniques often taught in childbirth education classes, the presence of a specialized labor coach (doula), water therapy, changing positions, acupuncture, and reflexology. During stage I of labor, pharmacologic pain management options include narcotics given IV or IM, epidural or spinal anesthesia. Epidural and spinal anesthesia may slow progress and prolong labor. They may also lead to maternal hypotension and fetal heart rate decelerations. During stage II of labor, anesthesia options include a pudendal block and local perineal anesthesia, especially prior to an episiotomy. Epidural and spinal anesthesia are not generally initiated during stage II.

<u>Induction of labor</u>
Induction of labor should be considered when there is evidence that continuing the pregnancy puts the mother, fetus, or both at risk. The most common reasons for inducing labor include post-dates pregnancy (>42 weeks gestation), signs of fetal distress, or maternal illness (e.g., preeclampsia). The method and likely success of different induction methods depends on several factors. These factors can be evaluated using the Bishop score. A cervical exam is performed and a score of 0 to 3 is given in the following areas: cervical position, consistency, effacement, dilation, and station. If the Bishop score is >6, IV Pitocin alone is sufficient. If the score is <6, a cervical ripening agent

should be used in addition to Pitocin to increase the likelihood of success. During induction procedures, continuous fetal monitoring is indicated.

Perineal lacerations

Perineal lacerations are a very common complication of vaginal delivery. Risk factors for developing perineal lacerations include first delivery, precipitous delivery, use of forceps or vacuum, shoulder dystocia, malpresentation, and fetal macrosomia. Lacerations are categorized as follows:

- First degree – laceration of vaginal mucosa.
- Second degree – laceration extends deep into vaginal tissue.
- Third degree – laceration extends into the external rectal sphincter muscle.
- Fourth degree – laceration goes through rectal mucosa.

Surgical repair is indicated. Complications of perineal lacerations include hemorrhage, chronic pain, difficulty passing bowel movements, urinary or fecal incontinence, and fistula formation.

UTI and asymptomatic bacteriuria during pregnancy

Pregnant women are at increased risk for developing urinary tract infections (UTIs) due to ureteral dilation, increased bladder volume, and decreased bladder tone. Approximately 5% of pregnancies are complicated by urinary tract infections. The incidence of asymptomatic bacteriuria is as high as 10%. Routine screening for UTI should be performed at the first prenatal visit and repeated during the third trimester. The risk of progressing to pyelonephritis is high (up to 50%), so all positive cultures should be treated. Cystitis can be treated with appropriate oral antibiotics. Pyelonephritis necessitates hospital admission and IV antibiotics. Follow-up cultures should be obtained. All women with group B strep bacteriuria should be given intrapartum antibiotic prophylaxis.

HIV positive pregnant women

All pregnant women should be offered screening for HIV infection. All HIV positive women should be given antiviral treatment in order to decrease the likelihood of transmitting HIV infection to the baby. Antiviral treatment should be administered regardless of CD4 cell count and viral load levels. The higher the maternal viral load, the more likely the transmission will occur. In general, it is recommended that HIV positive pregnant women receive aggressive antiviral treatment with multiple drugs. Most mother-to-child transmission occurs during delivery. Treatment with IV azidothymidine (AZT) during labor and delivery is recommended. C-section is recommended for women with a high viral load, or HIV positive women who have not received antiretroviral therapy. The newborn should be given anti-HIV therapy after birth. The mother should be counseled regarding breast-feeding and the risks of transmission. The usual regimen is six weeks of oral AZT. Both the mother and child should be seen by an HIV specialist.

Birth control

Oral contraceptives

Oral contraceptive pills (OCPs) can be either combined estrogen and progestin or progestin only. Combined OCPs have a >99% rate of effectiveness if used perfectly and an estimated 92% success rate with typical use. Contraindications to the use of combined OCPs include history of thromboembolic disease, cardiovascular disease, uncontrolled hypertension, heavy smoking, breast cancer, migraines, chronic liver disease, or any condition that leads to prolonged immobilization. Combined OCPs are not recommended for breast-feeding mothers. Progestin only OCPs are also effective. The only absolute contraindication is breast cancer; however, caution should be observed if a patient has any of the above conditions. Progestin only pills are considered safe for breast-feeding mothers and babies.

Intrauterine device

Intrauterine devices have an effectiveness rate of >99%. They do not prevent STDs. They are contraindicated in pregnancy, pelvic infection, gynecologic cancer, and breast cancer (hormone releasing IUD).

Condoms

Condoms are 85% effective with typical use and do provide protection against STDs.

Barriers

Vaginal barrier methods include the diaphragm, sponge, female condom, and cervical cap. They are all about 80% effective with typical use. The diaphragm and cervical cap must be fitted by a physician. The female condom and sponge are available over the counter. Spermicides are available over the counter and are generally used with a barrier.

Implants

Implants (Implanon®) are a progestin containing rod that is implanted subcutaneously. It lasts for three years and is >99% effective.

Sterilization

Both male and female sterilization procedures are available. Both tubal interruption surgery and vasectomy are >99% effective and considered permanent.

Elective abortion

Elective abortion is defined as the termination of pregnancy and removal of the embryo or fetus. Abortion is legal up to 24 weeks gestation. First trimester abortion is usually accomplished with a dilation and aspiration procedure. Post procedure antibiotics should be administered and complications are rare. First trimester abortions can also be performed with medication. Mifepristone (formerly RU-486) is effective up to a gestational age of 9 weeks. The patient should be administered the first dose in the physician's office and a second dose is taken at home. Significant bleeding and cramping can occur. The patient should have a follow-up visit in approximately 14 days to confirm complete termination of the pregnancy. Second trimester abortions are performed by dilation and evacuation. There is an increased morbidity and mortality associated with later abortions.

Sexually transmitted disease

Gonorrhea, *Chlamydia*, and trichomoniasis

Gonorrhea, *Chlamydia,* and trichomoniasis are all sexually transmitted infections. They are often asymptomatic, or patients may present with a history of a purulent vaginal discharge. Gonorrhea and *Chlamydia* cause a mucopurulent discharge and friable cervix. Both can lead to pelvic inflammatory disease. The diagnosis can be made using amplified DNA probe testing or culture. Treatment of gonorrhea is with ceftriaxone or cefixime. *Chlamydia* should be treated with a single dose of azithromycin 1 g PO for one dose OR by a 7-day course of doxycycline, 100 mg BID. Trichomoniasis typically causes a watery green-yellow vaginal discharge. The diagnosis is made by wet mount examination. The treatment is metronidazole.

Genital herpes and genital warts

Genital herpes can be caused by HSV-1 or HSV-2. Many patients are asymptomatic or may present with blisters and sores in the genital area. The diagnosis can be made by viral culture or Tzanck prep. There is no cure. Antiviral medication may reduce frequency and intensity of outbreaks. Daily antiviral medication may reduce risk of spread. Genital warts, also known as condylomata acuminata, appear as skin-colored papular "cauliflower" lesions on the genitalia and perineum. They are caused by human papillomavirus (HPV). The diagnosis is generally made clinically. Treatment includes topical medications. Imiquimod and podofilox can be applied by the patient. Trichloroacetic acid must be applied by a physician. Cryotherapy, electrocautery, and surgical excision are sometimes needed.

Syphilis and chancroid

Syphilis is a sexually transmitted disease caused by the bacteria *Treponema pallidum*. The incidence has increased with the emergence of AIDS. Primary syphilis presents with a painless genital ulcer or chancre. Secondary syphilis is characterized by a diffuse rash, fever, and generalized malaise. If untreated, the disease can progress to tertiary syphilis. Tertiary syphilis is characterized by neurologic and cardiac damage such as aortic aneurysms, aortic stenosis, meningitis, and dementia. Diagnosis is made by serology. A lumbar puncture is indicated if neurosyphilis is suspected. Treatment is with penicillin. Having untreated syphilis increases an individual's chance of contracting HIV. Chancroid is caused by the bacteria *Haemophilus ducreyi*. It generally presents as a painful genital ulcer. The size of the ulcer can vary from 3 to 50 mm. Treatment is with azithromycin, ceftriaxone, or ciprofloxacin. Untreated chancroid increases the risk of HIV transmission.

Vulvovaginitis

The most common cause is *Gardnerella*. Patients present with a history of a vaginal discharge that has a characteristic fishy odor. The diagnosis is made by the presence of "clue cells" on microscopic exam of a wet mount of the vaginal discharge. A KOH preparation is positive. Treatment is with metronidazole, either PO or topical. Vulvovaginitis can also be caused by *Candida* (yeast infection). Patients present with a history of vaginal itching and burning and a thick white discharge (with a "cottage cheese" appearance). A KOH preparation will show characteristic "budding" hyphae. Treatment is with intravaginal antifungals. Trichomonosis presents with a history of a profuse frothy green discharge. The diagnosis is made by the presence of motile trichomonads on wet mount. The treatment is with metronidazole.

Pediatric and Adolescent Medicine

Apgar score

The Apgar score was developed in 1952 by Dr. Virginia Apgar as a way to rapidly assess the health status of a newborn. The score is given at one and five minutes after birth. The score can be repeated at ten minutes and beyond if it remains low. A newborn is given a score of 0, 1, or 2 in five different categories: heart rate, respiratory effort, muscle tone, skin color, and reflex irritability. An Apgar score of eight or greater is considered normal. An Apgar score of less than three indicates a critically ill newborn. The five-minute Apgar score is considered more indicative of long-term prognosis.

Caput succedaneum, cephalhematoma, and subgaleal hemorrhage

Caput succedaneum, cephalhematoma, and subgaleal hemorrhage are possible abnormal findings on the newborn examination when examining the head of a newborn. Caput succedaneum is the presence of edema that crossed the suture lines. It is caused by trauma during the birth process. It is a benign condition that requires no treatment and resolves on its own during the first week of life. Cephalhematoma is characterized by a scalp swelling that does not cross the suture lines. It is caused by rupture of subperiosteal blood vessels due to trauma during delivery or as a complication of instrument assisted delivery. Jaundice and anemia are possible complications. Cephalhematomas usually resolve on their own; occasionally, phototherapy is needed to treat jaundice. Subgaleal hemorrhage is usually a complication of vacuum extraction. It presents as a boggy occipital mass that appears 12 to 72 hours after delivery. Subgaleal hemorrhage has the potential to lead to significant blood loss and should be monitored closely.

Down syndrome in newborns

Down syndrome, or trisomy 21, is one of the most common congenital abnormalities, with an incidence of approximately 1 in 700 births. The risk increases with increasing maternal age, especially after the age of 35 years. The diagnosis is suspected by the presence of certain physical features on the newborn exam. The following features are suggestive of Down syndrome: hypotonia, increased flexibility, redundant skin on the back of the neck, simian crease (single transverse palmar crease), slanted palpebral fissures, small and low set ears, flattened occiput, depressed nasal bridge, clinodactyly of the fifth finger, increased space between the first and second toes, and Brushfield's spots. The presence of six or more of these features on the newborn exam is highly suggestive of Down's syndrome and genetic studies should be performed.

Complications and management

There are numerous complications associated with Down syndrome. Cardiac problems include ventricular septal defects and endocardial cushion defects. Gastrointestinal abnormalities include duodenal atresia and Hirschsprung's disease. Individuals with Down syndrome have an increased risk of developing leukemia and Alzheimer's dementia. Down syndrome patients have moderate to severe mental retardation. Management of a Down syndrome patient requires a team approach. They should be evaluated and followed by a cardiologist, gastroenterologist, and developmental pediatrician. Physical and occupational therapy should also be part of the management plan. The average life expectancy is about 50 years of age.

Birth trauma

The most common traumatic complications of delivery include caput succedaneum, cephalhematoma, and subgaleal hemorrhage. Retinal and subconjunctival hemorrhages are also seen. Brachial plexus injury, including Erb-Duchenne paralysis (5th and 6th cervical nerve injury) and Klumpke paralysis (7th and 8th cervical nerve injury) are usually the result of excessive traction on the neck during a difficult delivery. Facial nerve injuries are sometimes seen. This is due to compression of the facial nerve against the mother's pelvis or injury from use of forceps. Fractures associated with delivery trauma include skull, clavicle, and extremity fracture. Clavicle fractures are the most common. Birth asphyxia can result from trauma of a complicated birth. This is often due to shoulder dystocia, cephalopelvic disproportion, or breech presentation.

Neonatal jaundice

Neonatal jaundice is very common, affecting up to 50% of newborns. The most common cause is physiologic jaundice. Other more serious causes include hemolysis, sepsis, and metabolic disorders. Physiologic jaundice is the result of indirect, unconjugated hyperbilirubinemia. Workup should include direct and indirect bilirubin, CBC, reticulocyte count, exam of peripheral blood smear and type, and Coombs test. It is generally a benign self-limited condition; however, there is a risk of kernicterus with very high bilirubin levels. Phototherapy is the treatment of choice for physiologic jaundice. The level at which to begin phototherapy depends on gestational age, weight of the newborn and age of neonate. The rate of rise of bilirubin levels should not exceed 5 mg/dL per day. In general, phototherapy should be considered in a term neonate who is 24 to 48 hours old and has a bilirubin <15 mg/dL. At a level of 20 mg/dL, exchange transfusion should be considered.

Neonatal sepsis

Neonatal sepsis is an overwhelming infection that occurs in the first month of life. Neonatal sepsis can be early onset (birth to 8 days) or late onset (8 to 28 days). Risk factors for early onset sepsis include prematurity, prolonged rupture of membranes, maternal fever during labor, and a history of group B strep colonization. Presenting symptoms include irritability, poor feeding, tachypnea, and temperature instability. The workup should be performed immediately and include CBC, blood culture, chest x-ray, U/A and culture, and CSF cell count and culture. Broad-spectrum antibiotic coverage (ampicillin and gentamicin) should be started, pending culture results. The most common pathogen is group B strep (GBS) followed by gram-negative rods. Late onset sepsis presents with similar symptoms. Pathogens include GBS, gram negatives, *S aureus*, *Enterococcus,* and *Pseudomonas*. The workup is the same as for early onset sepsis.

Transient tachypnea of the newborn

Transient tachypnea of the newborn (TTN) usually presents shortly after birth. The presenting symptoms are increased respiratory rate, often >60 breaths per minute. Risk factors include cesarean section, precipitous delivery, and maternal diabetes. Chest x-ray may show hyperinflation and prominent pulmonary vascular markings. Transient tachypnea of the newborn is usually self-limited and treatment is supportive care.

Meconium aspiration

Meconium aspiration occurs when a neonate aspirates meconium-stained fluid during delivery. The most significant risk factor is postdate delivery. If the infant appears healthy and vigorous at delivery, observation is sufficient. If the infant shows signs of distress, suctioning with an endotracheal tube is indicated. Meconium aspiration pneumonia is a very serious condition that requires NICU admission.

Hyaline membrane disease

Hyaline membrane disease, or infant respiratory distress syndrome, is seen in premature infants as the result of a lack of surfactant. Treatment involves respiratory support and surfactant administration via an endotracheal tube.

Chromosomal abnormalities

<u>Edward's, Patau's, Klinefelter's, and Turner's syndromes</u>

These syndromes are all chromosomal abnormalities. Edward's syndrome, or trisomy 18, affects approximately 1 in 6,000 live births. Most affected individuals die within the first year of life. The appearance is variable, but characteristic abnormalities include severe IUGR, severe mental retardation, and either clubfoot or "rocker-bottom feet." Patau's syndrome, or trisomy 13, affects approximately 1 in 6,000 births. Congenital abnormalities are severe and most die shortly after birth. Klinefelter's syndrome (XXY) occurs in approximately 1 in 1,000 births. Characteristics include mildly impaired IQ, gynecomastia, small testes, and decreased facial hair. Treatment includes testosterone replacement. Turner's syndrome (XO syndrome) occurs in 1 in 10,000 births. Characteristic findings include short stature, shield chest, webbed neck, coarctation of the aorta and amenorrhea. Therapy includes estrogen replacement.

Cystic fibrosis

Cystic fibrosis is an autosomal recessive disorder in which a defect in the CFTR protein (a chloride channel protein) leads to the production of abnormally thick, viscous mucous. It is one of the most common inherited diseases in the United States, affecting mostly individuals of Northern European decent. The diagnosis should be suspected in the newborn with meconium ileus. Other symptoms include frequent respiratory infections, failure to thrive, salty taste to the skin, and rectal prolapse. *Staphylococcus aureus* is the most common cause of pulmonary infection early in the disease; *Pseudomonas aeruginosa* is the dominant pathogen in more advanced cystic fibrosis. The diagnosis can be made by a sweat test or genetic testing. Prenatal testing and newborn screening tests are available. At this time, there is no cure for cystic fibrosis. Treatment is aimed at slowing the progression and alleviating symptoms. Treatments include mucolytic drugs, bronchodilators, antibiotics, and chest physiotherapy. Lung transplantation is sometimes an option for end-stage disease. Pancreatic enzyme replacement should be administered. End-stage lung disease is the most common cause of death. Life expectancy is 30 to 40 years.

Duchenne's muscular dystrophy

This is an x-linked recessive disorder. Duchenne's affects approximately 1 in 3,500 male births. Symptoms usually begin by the age of 5 years and start in the distal muscles and move proximally. Patients present with difficulty getting up and an unsteady waddling gait. Cardiomyopathy and mental impairment are late manifestations. Lab tests show an elevated creatinine kinase (CK). Diagnosis is made by muscle biopsy. Treatment involves physical therapy and braces. Most patients die by the age of 20 years.

Hemophilia

This is an x-linked recessive disorder. Hemophilia A (factor VIII deficiency) and hemophilia B (factor IX deficiency) are inherited disorders of coagulation. They occur in approximately 1 in

5,000 to 10,000 live births. Patients present with repeated episodes of spontaneous bleeding. Treatments include DDAVP for hemophilia A, replacement of clotting factors, and injury avoidance.

Pyloric stenosis

Pyloric stenosis is a condition caused by hypertrophy of the pylorus. It generally presents in the first 2 to 6 weeks of life with projectile nonbilious vomiting. It is more common in males, especially if they are the first-born. The diagnosis is made by history, palpation of an "olive" in the epigastric region, and the presence of peristaltic waves. Patients may also have signs of dehydration. The diagnosis is confirmed by ultrasound. An upper GI series may show a characteristic "string sign". Laboratory exam may show a hypokalemic, hypochloremic metabolic alkalosis. Treatment involves correcting the dehydration, alkalosis, and electrolyte abnormalities. Surgery needs to be performed as indicated and is curative.

Hirschsprung's disease

Hirschsprung's disease is a congenital disorder characterized by the absence of ganglion cells in the distal colon. Hirschsprung's disease occurs in about 1 in 5,000 births. It is more common in boys and in patients with Down syndrome. Patients usually present early in life with failure to pass meconium, vomiting, and abdominal distention. Mild cases can present later in childhood with constipation and poor weight gain. The diagnosis is suggested by abdominal x-ray showing a dilated proximal colon and absence of gas in the rectum. The diagnosis is confirmed by barium enema. The affected bowel segment will be narrowed and the proximal bowel will appear distended. Manometry and biopsy are also sometimes performed. Treatment is surgical removal of the aganglionic segment and subsequent pull-through of normal bowel.

Metatarsus varus

Metatarsus varus is sometimes seen on the newborn physical exam. It is also known as metatarsus adductus. On exam, the forefoot is twisted inward. It is often due to positioning of the foot in utero and does not require any treatment. On exam, it is critical to determine if the position is flexible and if the foot can be easily manipulated to the midline. If the position is fixed, treatment is required. Treatment options include corrective shoes, serial castings, and corrective bracing. Patients can sometimes also have hip dysplasia. With appropriate treatment, the prognosis is excellent.

Talipes equinovarus

Talipes equinovarus, or clubfoot, is a congenital structural foot deformity. It may be genetic. Patients present at birth with plantar flexion at the ankle, inversion of the heel, and medial deviation of the forefoot. The position is fixed. Treatment is serial casting or surgery.

Congenital hip dysplasia

Congenital hip dysplasia refers to abnormal hip joint formation leading to a hip that is either unstable or dislocated. Hip dysplasia occurs in about 3 to 4 per 1,000 live births. There is an increased incidence with a positive family history or breech presentation. It is more common in girls and occurs most commonly in the left hip. It can be unilateral or bilateral. Every newborn must be screened for hip dysplasia using Barlow's and Ortolani's maneuvers. Asymmetric thigh or buttock creases may be present. If dysplasia is suspected, an ultrasound should be obtained. The treatment of choice is a Pavlik harness.

Failure to thrive

Failure to thrive is defined as inadequate physical growth over a period of time. All children should have their height, weight, and head circumference (infants) plotted on a standard growth chart at each visit. If a child's measurements fall such that it crosses two percentile lines, than the child is said to be failing to thrive. Typically, a child's weight will show a decline first, followed by height. Head circumference is rarely involved. Etiologies can are divided into one of two categories: organic or nonorganic. When a child's height falls off their growth curve, the etiology is more likely to be organic. Nonorganic causes include psychosocial issues and inadequate feeding. There are numerous organic causes; almost any chronic disease can cause failure to thrive. The evaluation must include a thorough history and physical exam. Laboratory tests and further workup should be guided by the findings on the history and physical. Keeping a food diary and observing the parent-child interaction can sometimes be helpful. Occasionally, hospitalization is required.

Nutritional deficiencies

Scurvy

Scurvy refers to vitamin C deficiency. Presenting symptoms include bleeding from the gums and mucous membranes, poor healing, and failure to thrive. Treatment is vitamin C replacement.

Rickets

Rickets occurs when there is a vitamin D deficiency. Rickets can also occur as the result of inadequate calcium intake. A lack of sufficient vitamin D leads to inadequate calcium absorption, which will cause bone and muscle abnormalities. Treatment is vitamin D supplementation.

Kwashiorkor

Kwashiorkor is defined as an isolated protein deficiency. Patients present with a distended abdomen, edema, and failure to thrive. Treatment includes caloric supplementation with slow introduction of protein into the diet.

Marasmus

Marasmus is caused by a severe deficiency of all nutrients. Patients present with severe failure to thrive.

Vaccinations

HBV

The hepatitis B vaccine is a recombinant DNA vaccine. Universal vaccination of infants is recommended. The first dose is given in the hospital before the newborn is discharged, the second dose is given between 1 to 4 months, and the third dose is given between 6 to 18 months. All children eighteen and under should receive the three dose series if not previously immunized. The vaccine should be given to high-risk adults. The vaccine is contraindicated in people with a history of an allergic reaction to a previous dose of the vaccine.

DtaP

The vaccine against diphtheria, tetanus, and pertussis (acellular). The vaccine is made using small purified viral proteins. The vaccine series is begun in infants at 2 months of age. It is now recommended that children over the age of 11 years and adults 19 to 64 years receive a single booster dose of the new vaccine Tdap. The vaccine should not be given to an individual with a history of a serious allergic reaction or certain CNS abnormalities.

IPV

The inactivated polio vaccine is used almost exclusively in the United States. Oral polio vaccine (OPV) is used in countries where wild polio exists. The series is usually started at the two-month visit. The vaccine is contraindicated in individuals with a history of a severe allergic reaction to the antibiotics neomycin, streptomycin, or polymyxin B.

Hib

The Haemophilus influenzae type b (Hib) vaccine is given to all children under the age of 5 years, generally beginning at the two-month visit. Older children who have sickle cell disease, are asplenic, or are immunosuppressed from AIDS or cancer should also be vaccinated. The vaccine should not be given earlier that than 6 weeks of age or to individuals with a history of a significant allergic reaction to the vaccine.

MMR

The measles, mumps and rubella vaccine is a thimerosal-free live attenuated viral vaccine given in a two dose series generally at 15 months and at 4 to 6 years of age. The vaccine should not be administered to immunocompromised individuals or people with a history of a gelatin allergy. There is no scientific proof linking the MMR vaccine to the development of autism.

Varicella

The Varicella (chickenpox) vaccine is routinely administered at 12 to 18 months of age with a booster at age 4 to 6 years. The vaccine is contraindicated in individuals with allergies to gelatin, neomycin, or a previous dose of the vaccine. It should not be administered to pregnant women or people with T-cell immunodeficiency. The vaccine may not be administered for 5 months following a blood transfusion.

Influenza

The influenza vaccine is recommended annually for children 6 to 23 months of age, adults over the age of 50 years and most individuals with a chronic disease. It is recommended for all healthcare personnel and individuals living with a person at high-risk. It is also recommended before travel to certain areas of the world and before attending college, especially if residing in a dormitory. The vaccine is contraindicated in infants less than 6 months, people who are moderately to severely ill with a fever, and individuals with egg allergies. The nasal mist (live virus) form of the vaccine is contraindicated in children less than 2 years old, adults >50 years, people with a history of asthma or other chronic disease, and pregnant women.

Meningococcal

The meningococcal vaccine is currently recommended for children at age 11 to 12 years and before starting high school. It is also recommended before college entry and for military recruits. It is contraindicated in individuals with a latex allergy or hypersensitivity to diphtheria toxoid.

Iron deficiency anemia

Iron deficiency anemia is common and routine screening is recommended for all children at 9 to 15 months, with additional screening recommended for at-risk children. Iron deficiency anemia can result from inadequate intake or from blood loss. Premature infants and infants and toddlers that consume large quantities of cow's milk are at high risk. A history of pica increases the risk of iron deficiency anemia. A hemoglobin of <11 g/dL is considered abnormal. The treatment involves iron replacement. Follow-up CBC should be performed. If anemia does not resolve, further workup in indicated.

Lead poisoning

Lead poisoning in children remains a common problem. The most common source is exposure to lead paint, which is usually found in homes built before 1950. Contaminated water from lead containing pipes is also a source. Universal screening of children at ages 9 to 12 months is recommended in most communities. Communities with low rates of elevated lead levels in children and a low percentage of homes built before 1950 may be able to do targeted screening. Children at high risk should be initially screened at 6 months. Subsequent screening depends on the initial lead level. A level of >10 mcg/dL is considered abnormal. A careful history should be performed to determine the source of the lead exposure. Counseling the topics of dietary measures, increasing iron, vitamin C and calcium, and avoidance of lead paint should be performed. Acute lead poisoning or levels >45 mcg/dL may require chelation therapy.

Enuresis

Enuresis is a very common problem in children. Primary enuresis is defined as the condition of never having been dry at night. Secondary enuresis is when a child resumes bed-wetting after a period of being dry of at least 6 months. Enuresis is more common in boys. The family must be reassured that the problem is very common and most patients will outgrow bed-wetting before the age of 12 years. A screening urinalysis should be performed. Treatment is usually just reassurance. In older children who are bothered by the bed-wetting, treatment options include different types of alarm systems to wake a child upon wetting the bed. Medications that are used include DDAVP, imipramine, and oxybutynin.

Strabismus

Strabismus is term that describes misalignment of the eyes. Esotropia describes strabismus when the eyes look inward; exotropia is when the eyes look outward. All infants should be screened for strabismus as part of the newborn exam. This can be performed with either the cover test (when the dominant eye is covered, the weaker eye will focus on a particular object) or Hirschberg test (when a light is shined in the patient's eyes the reflection will not appear in the same spot). Most strabismus detected in newborns is benign and resolves in the first few months of life. If the strabismus is fixed, the infant should be referred to an ophthalmologist for evaluation. Strabismus can be caused by a central nervous system disorder of or from an extraocular muscle problem. Treatment options include eye patching and surgery.

Slipped capital femoral epiphysis

Slipped capital femoral epiphysis occurs when a growth plate abnormality leads to displacement of the femoral head from the hip joint. It typically affects children ages 11 to 16 years. Boys are affected more often than girls, particularly if they are overweight. Patients present with pain and limp. The diagnosis is made by x-ray. Treatment is surgical pinning.

Leg-Calve-Perthes disease

Legg-Calve-Perthes disease is also known as avascular necrosis of the femoral head. It is typically seen in children ages 4 to 8 years; it is more common in boys. Patients present with pain, limp, and decreased range of motion. Diagnosis is made by x-ray. Treatment is rest and anti-inflammatory medications.

Osgood-Schlatter syndrome

Osgood-Schlatter syndrome is an overuse syndrome where patients present with pain and tenderness over the tibial tuberosity. It typically presents in adolescent athletes. Treatment is rest and pain management. The condition is benign and generally resolves in time.

Autism

Autism is a developmental disorder characterized by impaired social interactions and communication abnormalities. Autism is part of a spectrum of disorders known as autism spectrum disorders (ASD) ranging in severity from mild language and behavioral deficits to a complete inability to communicate. Patients are typically diagnosed between 1 to 3 years of age when they present with delayed language skills, lack of interpersonal interactions, and abnormal behaviors. Abnormal behaviors can include repetitive movements like rocking or specific routines or rituals. The cause is still unknown. No study has proven a link between MMR vaccination and autism. It is more common in boys and there appears to be a genetic component. Treatment includes behavioral and communication therapies.

Review Video: Autism
Visit mometrix.com/academy and enter code: 395410

Attention-deficit hyperactivity disorder

ADHD is a commonly diagnosed disorder characterized by inattentiveness, hyperactivity, and impulsivity. In order to be diagnosed with ADHD, a child must exhibit six or more symptoms from at least two of the categories. The symptoms must be present at both home and school. The Conners' ADHD Index and symptom scales are useful in making the diagnosis. Attention-deficit hyperactivity disorder is typically diagnosed early in childhood, but the disorder also exists in adults. The cause is unknown and there does appear to be a hereditary component. It is more common in boys. It can be associated with other psychiatric disorders such as depression, conduct disorders, and anxiety disorders. Treatment includes medications (stimulants), behavior modification, and psychotherapy.

Croup

Croup is a viral upper respiratory infection typically diagnosed in children between the ages of 6 months and 3 years. It is most prevalent in the fall and winter. Typical presentation is a low-grade fever and gradual onset of respiratory distress characterized by inspiratory and expiratory stridor. A chest x-ray may show the characteristic steeple sign. Treatment includes humidified oxygen (croup tent), steroids, and racemic epinephrine.

Epiglottitis

Epiglottitis is a bacterial infection of the epiglottis. The most common pathogens are strep, staph, and *H influenzae*. Presenting symptoms include rapid onset of high fever and difficulty breathing. Patients are often leaning forward and drooling. Lateral neck x-ray may show a "thumbprint sign". Epiglottitis is a life-threatening emergency and the first priority is to secure an airway. This is sometimes performed under anesthesia. Intravenous antibiotics are indicated.

Febrile seizures

Febrile seizures are a common occurrence in childhood. They usually occur in children between the ages of 6 months and 5 years who have rectal temperatures >102° F. A simple febrile seizure is generalized, lasts <15 minutes and does not occur more than once during a 24 hour period. Complex febrile seizures may be focal, last >15 minutes or occur more than once in a 24-hour period. Simple febrile seizures generally do not need a workup. Parents should be counseled about fever control and the possibility of the child having another febrile seizure. Frequent recurrences of febrile seizure may require use of antiseizure medication. Complex febrile seizures require a complete neurologic workup, including a lumbar puncture.

Heart murmurs

Heart murmurs are common findings on the pediatric physical exam and approximately 40% are benign. A murmur is more likely benign if it is soft, systolic, and short in duration. The patient should not have any other symptoms of cardiac disease and there should be a normal S1 and S2 on cardiac auscultation. The quality of functional murmurs often changes when a patient changes position from lying to sitting or standing. The presence of failure to thrive, exercise intolerance, or cyanosis are all indications that cardiac disease is present. Still's murmur is a common functional murmur of childhood. It is a soft systolic murmur heard best along the left sternal border. It generally disappears as a child grows. Any suspicion that heart murmur is pathologic requires referral to a cardiologist.

Kawasaki's disease

Kawasaki's disease, also known as mucocutaneous lymph node syndrome, is an inflammatory childhood disease of unknown etiology. It typically affects children younger than 5 years of age and is more common in boys. In order for the diagnosis to be made, fever must be present for at least 5 days and the patient must exhibit at least four of the following symptoms: bilateral conjunctivitis, inflammation of the oral mucosa including cracked lips and strawberry tongue, cervical lymphadenopathy, rash and redness, swelling, and ultimately peeling of the hands and feet. The diagnosis is made clinically and the treatment is with aspirin and IVIG. The most serious complication is coronary artery aneurysm. The patient must be examined and followed by a cardiologist.

Sexual development

Tanner staging is a system used to describe the stages of sexual development. The stages are as follows:

- Tanner I – prepubescent, no signs of sexual development.
- Tanner II – sparse pubic hair, enlargement of scrotum and testes, breast buds.
- Tanner III – darker, coarser, more curled pubic hair, enlargement of penis in length, enlargement and elevation of breast and areola.
- Tanner IV – pubic hair resembles adult with more limited distribution, increase in length and breadth of penis and darkening of scrotal skin, areola and papilla form secondary mound.
- Tanner V – mature.

Onset of puberty is between ages 9 to 13 years for boys and 8 to 13 years for girls. Signs of puberty at younger ages are considered precocious and should be investigated. Lack of signs of puberty by age 13 years warrants a workup.

Acne vulgaris

Acne vulgaris is caused by blockage of the pilosebaceous unit. It is extremely common, affecting approximately 85% of teenagers and young adults. Acne is generally divided by degree of severity. Acne is considered mild if there are fewer than 30 total lesions with few inflammatory lesions. Mild acne is generally treated with a topical benzoyl peroxide preparation, a topical antibiotic, or sometimes a mild topical Retin-A® preparation at night. Moderate acne can have up to 100 to 125 total lesions with a higher proportion being inflammatory. Moderate acne is frequently treated with an oral antibiotic as well as topical preparation. Severe acne is characterized by >125 lesions, many inflammatory lesions and the presence of cysts. Severe acne is often treated with oral isotretinoin (Accutane®). If Accutane is used, LFTs must be followed and girls must be counseled regarding the teratogenicity of the medication.

Acute otitis media

Acute otitis media (AOM) is one of the most common diagnoses made in pediatrics. Children between the ages of 6 months and 3 years are most commonly affected. Risk factors include attendance at a group day care facility, exposure to smoke and air pollution, and a positive family history. Infants who drink from a bottle in a supine position are at increased risk. Acute otitis media often develops as a complication of a viral upper respiratory infection. Approximately 25% of AOM are viral. Common bacterial pathogens include *Streptococcus pneumoniae*, *Haemophilus influenzae* and *Moraxella catarrhalis*. The diagnosis is made clinically. Pain medication and observation is an appropriate therapeutic approach in children older than 6 months. Appropriate antibiotic choices include amoxicillin, Augmentin®, Bactrim®, and second-generation cephalosporins.

General Surgery

Acute abdomen

Acute abdomen is defined as the acute onset of severe abdominal pain. There are many possible causes of acute abdomen. It often requires surgical intervention. Patients can present with abdominal pain, fever, nausea, vomiting, diarrhea, or constipation. The physical exam may be significant for a patient who appears ill and has a tender, rigid abdomen. The physical exam should check for guarding, rebound, and the presence and quality of bowel sounds. A rectal exam is an essential part of the workup. The workup should include CBC, electrolytes, BUN/creatinine, LFTs, amylase, and lipase. All women of childbearing age should have a pregnancy test. Chest x-ray, abdominal x-ray, ultrasound, and CT can all be helpful in making the diagnosis. Surgical consultation and exploratory laparotomy are sometimes necessary.

Acute appendicitis

Acute appendicitis is one of the most common causes of acute abdomen. It is thought to be caused by obstruction of the appendix eventually leading to necrosis and perforation. A classic presentation is a history of periumbilical pain that migrated to the right lower quadrant. Only about 50% of patients present with classic symptoms. The onset of pain is often followed by nausea, vomiting, anorexia, and a low-grade fever. The exam may be significant for RLQ tenderness, guarding and rebound. Patients may have a positive psoas sign, obturator sign, or Rovsing's sign. Laboratory exam may show leukocytosis. The diagnosis can usually be made clinically; however, CT, abdominal x-ray or ultrasound may be helpful. Treatment is appendectomy. Complications include perforation, peritonitis, abscess, and pylephlebitis.

Bowel obstruction

A bowel obstruction refers to complete or partial blockage of the intestine. The numerous causes of bowel obstruction include tumors, adhesions from prior surgery, foreign bodies, hernias, and fecal impaction. Patients usually present with abdominal pain, vomiting, diverticular disease, and constipation. They may have fever and signs of dehydration. The physical exam may show a tender, distended abdomen, peristaltic waves, and high-pitched tinkling bowel sounds. The workup should include CBC, electrolytes, abdominal x-ray, and possibly a CT scan. The patient should be NPO and an NG tube should be placed. Further management depends on the degree of obstruction and the specific cause. Antibiotics and surgery are often required.

Diverticular disease

Diverticular disease is very common in individuals over the age of 40 years. It is estimated that 50% of people over the age of 50 years have diverticula. Diverticulosis is the presence of diverticula, and diverticulitis is inflammation or infection of diverticula. Patients with diverticulosis are generally asymptomatic, often presenting with LLQ abdominal pain. Nausea, vomiting, constipation, and diarrhea may also be present. On physical exam, the patient may have a fever, LLQ abdominal tenderness or mass and abdominal distention. A CT scan with IV and oral contrast is the best study for making the diagnosis. Management includes making the patient NPO and placing an NG tube. Broad-spectrum IV antibiotics should be started. Surgery is indicated for recurrent disease or to treat complications such as perforation or obstruction.

Hemorrhoids

Hemorrhoids are swollen, inflamed veins of the anus and rectum. They often develop because of increased pressure in the lower rectum from chronic constipation or pregnancy. Patients often present with pain, itching, and bright red streaks of blood on the stool or toilet tissue. The diagnosis is generally made by observation of the hemorrhoids on physical exam. Anoscopy is sometimes helpful to diagnose internal hemorrhoids. Treatment includes management of symptoms with pain medications and topical anti-inflammatory creams. Management should also include dietary measures to alleviate constipation. Persistent, bleeding hemorrhoids or thrombosed hemorrhoids may require more invasive treatment such as rubber band ligation, sclerosis, or surgical excision.

Hernias

Inguinal and umbilical hernias

Inguinal hernias are the most common in adults and second most common hernia in children. They can be due to a congenital abnormality or result from strain or injury. Patients present with pain and swelling in the groin area. About 8% to 10% are bilateral. The diagnosis is made by physical exam and the treatment is surgery. Umbilical hernias are the most common type of hernia in children. Infants present with a bulging umbilicus when crying or staining. Most umbilical hernias close on their own by age 1 year. If not closed by age 4 years, surgery may be indicated.

Femoral, incisional, and epigastric hernias

Femoral hernias occur because of a weakness in the femoral canal. They are more common in women than in men. Patients present with swelling in the groin or upper thigh. Complications such as incarceration and strangulation are common and surgical repair is indicated. Incisional hernias occur at the incisional site of a previous surgery. They can be the result of excessive tension placed when closing an incision. Surgery with revision of the incision may be needed. Epigastric hernias are caused by weakness in the upper abdominal wall. They can become incarcerated. Treatment is surgery.

Breast cancer

Breast cancer is the second leading cause of cancer death in women. The most common presentation is a palpable lump in the breast. All breast lumps should be observed until a definitive diagnosis is made. Characteristics of a lump due to fibrocystic disease include a painful mass and changes in the mass related to the menstrual cycle. Fibrocystic disease is benign. All cysts should be evaluated with needle aspiration, which may be both diagnostic and curative. Solid masses should be evaluated with a mammogram, followed by either needle biopsy or excisional biopsy. Treatment depends on stage and cell type. Treatment generally includes surgery, either lumpectomy or mastectomy, and chemotherapy. Hormone therapy is effective in tumors that are estrogen-receptor or progesterone-receptor positive.

Geriatric Medicine

Dementia

Dementia is a progressive neurologic disorder characterized by impaired memory and cognitive abilities. The two main types of dementia are Alzheimer's disease and vascular dementia. Alzheimer's dementia is the most common. Patients with dementia present with progressive confusion, memory loss, and increasing difficulties with daily living activities. The diagnosis is made by history and physical exam. Other, potentially reversible, causes of dementia must be ruled out. Patients should have a CBC, LFT, TFT, and have their electrolyte, glucose, and vitamin B12 levels checked. Imaging studies may be indicated if intracranial bleeds or tumors are suspected. The mini-mental status exam (MMSE) should be administered to assess cognitive ability. Treatment options include cholinesterase inhibitors, N-methyl-D-aspartate (NMDA) antagonists, and vitamin E. Antipsychotic and antidepressant medication may be helpful.

Lewy body dementia vs. Alzheimer's dementia

Lewy body dementia is a form of dementia characterized by the presence of Lewy bodies. Lewy bodies are aggregates of protein that are seen inside nerve cells. They are seen in both Parkinson's disease and Lewy body dementia. Patients with Lewy body dementia often have fluctuating symptoms and are more likely to hallucinate than Alzheimer's patients. Patients with Lewy body dementia may also have Parkinson's-like symptoms. The diagnosis is made by history, physical exam, and mental status evaluation. Treatment options include cholinesterase inhibitors, Parkinson's medications, antidepressants, and antipsychotic medications. Behavioral management is important with memory aids and providing structure and routine. Patients with Lewy body dementia require close observation and daily care because of their unpredictability.

Delirium

Delirium is an acute change in mental status and can be distinguished from dementia by its rapid and sudden onset. Patients present with the rapid onset of confusion and inability to communicate clearly and rationally. Hyperactive delirium is characterized by agitation and combativeness. Patients with hypoactive delirium are quiet and non-communicative. Delirium is very common in elderly hospitalized patients, affecting as many as 30% to 40%. The workup for delirium should include a complete history and physical exam. Laboratory tests and imaging studies should be performed to rule out any possible underlying cause. Treatment options include low-dose antipsychotics such as haloperidol. Benzodiazepines can be used to treat agitation. It is often helpful for the delirious patient to have family members or other familiar individuals present to help orient them.

Parkinson's disease

Parkinson's disease is a progressive degenerative central nervous system disorder that primarily affects movement. Parkinson's disease is caused by the loss of dopamine containing neurons in the substantia nigra. Parkinson's disease is more common in older individuals and in men. Heredity may play a small role. The classic presenting symptoms are a resting, pill-rolling tremor, bradykinesia, and cogwheel rigidity. Patients may also have impaired balance, inability to blink or smile that leads to a blank stare appearance, and signs of dementia. The diagnosis is made clinically. Other potential causes such as drug toxicity or trauma should be ruled out. The first choice of treatment is Sinemet®. Sinemet® is a combination of levodopa and carbidopa. Carbidopa blocks the peripheral breakdown of levodopa, allowing more of the drug to cross the blood-brain barrier and to be converted to dopamine. Other treatment options include dopamine agonists, monoamine oxidase type B (MAO-B) inhibitors, catechol-O-methyltransferase (COMT) inhibitors, anticholinergics, and antiviral medications. Physical therapy is important to help maintain as much function as possible. Deep brain stimulation via surgical electrode implantation can also be used for advanced cases.

Review Video: Parkinson's Disease
Visit mometrix.com/academy and enter code: 110876

Incontinence

Urge incontinence

Urinary incontinence is the involuntary loss of urine. There are several types of urinary incontinence in geriatric patients and urge incontinence is the most common type. It is characterized by a sudden intense urge to urinate followed by loss of urine. This occurs frequently and often at night. The diagnosis is made by measuring post-void residual, which will be >200 mL. Workup should include a urinalysis (U/A) and culture to rule out urinary tract infection (UTI). Urge incontinence can be caused by multiple sclerosis (MS) or Parkinson's disease. It can also be associated with Alzheimer's disease. Treatment options include pelvic muscle strengthening, bladder training, reducing caffeine, and scheduling frequent bathroom trips. Drug treatments include anticholinergics, oxybutynin, tolterodine, and nortriptyline.

Stress incontinence

Stress incontinence is the involuntary loss or urine when increased pressure is placed on the bladder. This can occur with sneezing, coughing, laughing, heavy lifting, or during exercise. Stress incontinence is much more common in women and is due to weakening of the pelvic floor muscles. Risk factors include advanced age, history of multiple deliveries, and obesity. Patients present with a history of involuntary urination during sneezing, coughing, laughing, etc. The diagnosis is generally made by history. Urinary tract infection should be ruled out. A urinary stress test is sometimes performed. Treatment options include pelvic floor muscle exercises, limiting caffeine and fluid consumption, pads and urethral plugs, and pelvic surgery.

Overflow incontinence

Overflow incontinence is characterized by a continuous leak of small amounts of urine. It is most often seen in men and is due to enlargement of the prostate. It can also be caused by obstruction of the bladder due to tumors or scar tissue, neurologic damage and medications such as anticholinergics, calcium channel blockers, and narcotics. The diagnosis is made by history and physical exam. Post-void residual will generally be greater than 450 mL. Urodynamic testing can be helpful in determining the cause. Acute urinary retention may require bladder catheterization. Alpha-blockers are used to relax the internal sphincter.

Osteoporosis

Osteoporosis is a chronic bone disorder in which bone mineral density is reduced, leading to an increased risk of pathologic fractures. Risk factors for developing osteoporosis include age, female sex, family history, and having a small frame. Medications that increase the risk include steroids and thyroid hormone. Having a sedentary lifestyle, alcoholism, and inadequate calcium intake also increase the risk of osteoporosis. The longer a patient is exposed to estrogen (early menarche or late menopause), the lower the risk of developing osteoporosis. Patients often present with pathologic fractures of the spine or hip. Patients may have a history of height loss. The diagnosis is made by dual energy x-ray absorptiometry (DEXA), which measures bone density. The severity of the disease can be measured using T-scores, which compare bone density values to those of healthy young adults. Z-scores compare bone density values to age- and sex-matched controls. Treatment options include increasing dietary calcium, exercise, and smoking cessation. Medications used to treat osteoporosis include bisphosphonates, selective estrogen receptor modulators (SERMs), calcitonin, and parathyroid hormone.

Benign prostatic hypertrophy

Benign prostatic hypertrophy refers to the enlargement of the prostate gland that often accompanies aging. Many men with BPH are asymptomatic. When the prostate becomes large enough, it can obstruct urine flow, leading to symptoms including urinary frequency, nocturia, weak urinary stream, difficulty emptying the bladder, and difficulty with the initiation of voiding. An enlarged prostate can sometimes be detected on rectal exam. Serum PSA and post-void residual volume should be checked. Transrectal ultrasound and biopsy may be needed to rule out prostate cancer. Medical treatments include alpha-blockers and 5α-reductase inhibitors. Both medications act to shrink the prostate and can be used together. Transurethral resection of the prostate (TURP) and prostatectomy are sometimes indicated.

Emergency Medicine

Shock

Shock is defined as an emergency medical condition in which the circulatory system is unable to meet the oxygen delivery needs of the body. Shock is a medical emergency that if left untreated, can lead to irreversible organ damage and death. Shock is divided into three categories based on the etiology: hypovolemic, cardiogenic, and distributive (septic). Some of the more common causes of shock include trauma, ruptured aneurysm, cardiac failure, and sepsis. The presenting signs of shock include tachycardia, tachypnea, cool clammy skin, altered mental status, and hypotension. First attention must be given to evaluating and managing the ABCs (airway, breathing, and circulation). Intravenous access must be established. It is generally recommended that two large bore IV catheters be placed. Administer oxygen, evaluate respiratory status, and consider intubation. The cause of shock should be investigated. Work up should include CBC, metabolic panel, toxicology screen, arterial blood gas, and chest x-ray. Once the etiology is established, it should be treated. Use of pressers such as epinephrine, dopamine, and dobutamine should be considered.

Toxic ingestions

There are many toxic substances that can potentially be ingested. Signs and symptoms, as well as a treatment regimen, depend on identifying the substance. General management principles can be applied to most ingestions. The use of ipecac to induce vomiting is ineffective for treatment of ingestions and is no longer recommended. Gastric lavage is generally considered useful if it can be done within 1.5 hours of the ingestion. The airway must be protected during lavage. Patients with depressed mental status require intubation. Activated charcoal should be given as soon as possible. Some specific antidotes for ingestions include: N-acetylcysteine for acetaminophen, physostigmine for anticholinergics, hyperbaric oxygen for carbon monoxide, deferoxamine for iron, and ethylenediamine tetraacetic acid (EDTA) for lead.

Myocardial infarction

Myocardial infarction occurs when there is inadequate blood supply to a portion of the myocardium. Risk factors for myocardial infarction include smoking, hypertension, elevated lipid levels, diabetes, and obesity. The most common cause is blockage of the coronary arteries from atherosclerosis. Myocardial infarction can also be due to coronary artery spasm. Patients classically complain of substernal pressure. The pain may radiate to the back or down the left arm. Patients may have shortness of breath, diaphoresis, nausea, and vomiting. The diagnosis is generally confirmed by EKG changes and the presence of elevated cardiac enzymes. Initial emergency room management includes stabilizing the ABCs (airway, breathing, and circulation). In appropriate medical centers, percutaneous coronary intervention (PCI) is the treatment of choice if it can be started within ninety minutes. Thrombolytic therapy is appropriate if PCI is not available. Treatment should also include morphine for pain, oxygen, and anticoagulation. Complications include arrhythmias, heart failure, and death.

Acute appendicitis

Appendicitis is a condition characterized by the obstruction and inflammation of the appendix. Appendicitis is one of the most common causes of acute abdominal pain. The classic presentation is a history of periumbilical pain that migrates to the right lower quadrant usually over a period of hours. Patients frequently complain of fever, anorexia, nausea, and vomiting. Physical exam may be significant for tenderness over McBurney's point, a positive psoas or obturator sign, guarding, and rebound tenderness. Patients usually try to remain still since movements generally elicit pain. Laboratory exam may be significant for a leukocytosis. The diagnosis is generally made clinically. Ultrasound or CT scan can help confirm the diagnosis. Treatment is surgical removal of the appendix.

Hyperthermia

Hyperthermia is defined as a condition in which the body produces or absorbs more heat than it can eliminate. Heat exhaustion is the milder form of hyperthermia and it is characterized by a mild increase in body temperature and dehydration. Heat stroke is a severe condition in which the body temperature rises above 41.1°C. Heat stroke is associated with a high mortality rate. The symptoms of hyperthermia include fatigue, nausea, vomiting, and an altered mental status. Physical exam is significant for tachycardia, tachypnea, and an elevated body temperature. It is a medical emergency. Treatment includes rapid cooling measures with ice pack and water immersion and IV hydration.

Hypothermia

Hypothermia is defined as the core body temperature <35°C. It occurs when the body is unable to produce sufficient heat to make up for losses. The risk of hypothermia is increased at both ends of the age spectrum. Alcohol, drug use, and conditions that cause mental impairment, such as Alzheimer's disease or psychiatric illness, also increase the risk of hypothermia. Patients usually present with shivering, confusion, slurred speech, and clumsiness. The diagnosis is confirmed by the presence of a low core body temperature. Treatment involves rewarming the patient. Heat blankets, heat packs, warmed IV saline, and warmed humidified oxygen are all used. Patients may appear dead, but should not be considered dead until their core body temperature has been returned to normal.

Burns

Burns are defined as injury to the skin caused by heat, cold, radiation, chemicals, electricity, or friction. Burns are generally classified by their severity. First-degree burns, or partial thickness burns, only involve the epidermis. They are characterized by erythema and mild pain. Second-degree burns involve the dermis. They can be superficial or deep. They are characterized by erythema, significant pain, and blistering. Third-degree burns, or full thickness burns, are characterized by areas that appear charred, dry, or white. There is often no pain. Subcutaneous tissue may be involved. Patients must also be evaluated for the extent of burns. This is usually done using the rule of nines. Superficial burns may be managed on an outpatient basis with dressings, wound care, and pain management. Severe burns require hospital admission. Emergency care involves establishment of the ABCs (airway, breathing, and circulation), IV fluids, and topical care with silver sulfadiazine and sterile dressings.

Head trauma

Head trauma is one of the most common causes of death in young people. The most common causes are motor vehicle accidents, falls, sports-related injuries, and assaults. Head injuries can be divided into two main categories, closed and penetrating. The Glasgow Coma Scale (GCS) is an important tool used to assess the clinical status of head injury patients. The scale rates patients in the areas of eye opening, motor response, and verbal response. Signs and symptoms of head trauma include loss of consciousness, headaches, nausea, vomiting, and focal neurologic deficits.

Cerebral spinal fluid leakage, Battle's sign, hemotympanum and raccoon eyes are all signs of a basilar skull fracture. A GCS score of 15 is indicative of a mild head injury. A score of 14 or less is indicative of a more severe injury. The diagnosis is generally made by history, physical exam, and head CT. Cervical spine injury must always be ruled out. Management includes establishment of ABCs (airway, breathing, and circulation), hyperventilation if increased intracranial pressure is present, and neurosurgical consultation.

Preventative Medicine/Public Health

Types of prevention

Primary

Primary prevention describes measures undertaken to avoid the development of disease. There are many examples of primary prevention, including: immunizations, counseling high-risk behavior, and prophylactic medicines.

Secondary

Secondary prevention is action taken to prevent the progression of a disease. This includes early detection, as in cancer screening, HIV screening, and blood pressure monitoring.

Tertiary

Tertiary prevention is aimed at minimizing damage and complications from a particular disease. Examples of tertiary prevention include cancer chemotherapy, antihypertensive medication, insulin for blood glucose control in diabetics, and renal dialysis.

Cancer screening guidelines

The following are recommended cancer screening procedures:

- Cervical cancer – Annual PAP tests for all women within 3 years onset of sexual activity and not later than age 21 years. Women over the age of 70 years who have had 3 consecutive normal PAP tests no longer require screening. Women who have had a total hysterectomy do not require screening.
- Breast cancer – Yearly mammograms should be performed beginning at the age of 40 years. Breast self-exam should be taught to women beginning in their twenties.
- Colon cancer – Patients over the age of 50 years should have annual screening for occult blood in the stool and sigmoidoscopy every 3 to 5 years or colonoscopy every 10 years. Patients with a family history of colon cancer should begin screening at the age of 40 years.
- Prostate cancer – Digital rectal exam and prostate-specific antigen (PSA) annually beginning at age 50 years. High-risk men (African-American or positive family history) should be screened beginning at age 40 years.
- Skin cancer – Patients should be counseled regarding suspicious skin lesions and receive a skin exam every 3 years. Patients should also be advised about the importance of using sunscreen.
- Testicular cancer – All men should receive an annual testicular exam by a physician. Patients should be taught and encouraged to do testicular self-exam.
- Ovarian cancer – There is no recommended screening procedure for ovarian cancer.

Adult immunizations

The following vaccines are recommended for adults:

- Tetanus and diphtheria – give primary series if not performed in childhood, followed by boosters every 10 years.
- Measles, mumps, rubella – Patients born after 1957 and not previously immunized should be given two doses a minimum of 1 month apart.

- Influenza – Yearly vaccine is recommended for patients over the age of 50 years or patients at risk for severe disease. This includes immunocompromised patients and patients with chronic disease.
- Pneumococcal – All patients over the age of 65 years, or high-risk patients over the age of 50 years.
- Varicella – Should be given to all adults with without evidence of immunity. Two doses should be administered 4 to 8 weeks apart.
- Human papilloma virus (HPV) – Three dose series should be given to all women <26 years of age who have not been previously immunized.
- Meningococcal -- All asplenic adults and first-year college students who will be living in a dormitory.
- Herpes zoster – All adults over the age of 60 years.
- Hepatitis A and B – Recommended for patients at risk due to lifestyle, occupation, or travel plans.

Smoking cessation methods

Smoking is the leading cause of preventable death in the United States today. The benefits of quitting are well-established. Nicotine is addictive and smoking cessation leads to symptoms of withdrawal. This issue should be addressed by the primary care physician. The Public Health Service recommends the 4-A's approach to aid patients with smoking cessation:

- Asking – about smoking.
- Advice – how to approach quitting and setting a date to quit.
- Assistance – with counseling as well as pharmacologic aids. Counseling options include smoking cessation groups and hypnosis. Drugs available to help with smoking cessation include nicotine replacement products available as patches, gum, nasal spray, and inhalers. Bupropion is an antidepressant used to aid in smoking cessation. It is contraindicated in patients with a history of seizures. Counseling must include the possibility of weight gain and advice about diet and exercise.
- Arranging – a follow-up appointment 2 to 4 weeks after the date set for quitting.

The combination of counseling and support groups with drug therapy has a smoking cessation success rate of about 50%.

Travel prophylaxis for malaria

Specific prophylaxis for travel depends on the individual patient's health status and the travel destination. If a patient is traveling to a country with a risk of malaria, appropriate prophylaxis must be prescribed. Depending on the level of risk of the particular country, prophylaxis may include taking precautions to avoid mosquito bites, as well as different combinations of antimalarial drugs. The drugs used for malarial prophylaxis include mefloquine, doxycycline, Malarone, chloroquine, and proguanil. The specific regimen depends on the type of malaria and the resistance patterns of the location to be traveled. Mosquito bite avoidance is about 85% effective and chemoprophylaxis is about 75% to 95% effective in preventing malaria. A patient frequently does not exhibit symptoms of malaria until returning home.

Reporting to the health department

The requirement for reporting diseases to the state health department varies by state, but most states require reporting of the following:

- Animal bites requiring rabies prophylaxis
- Anthrax
- Botulism
- Brucellosis
- Cholera
- Diphtheria
- Encephalitis
- Glanders
- Hantavirus
- Hepatitis A in a food handler
- Measles, mumps or rubella
- Severe acute respiratory syndrome (SARS)
- Meningococcemia
- Rabies
- Smallpox
- Syphilis
- Tuberculosis
- Typhoid

Other diseases may mandate reporting and a physician should be aware of the requirements of the state in which they are practicing.

Incidence and prevalence

Incidence is defined as the number of new cases of a disease that develop over a certain period of time in a population that is at risk for developing the disease. Incidence is a measure of risk. It is calculated as follows:

Incidence per 1,000 = [(Number of new cases during time period) / (total number of persons at risk)] x 1,000

Prevalence is defined as the number of cases that currently exist at a specified time. Prevalence is not a measure of risk. Prevalence is influenced by the duration of a disease. Therapies that prolong the survival of patients with a particular disease will increase the prevalence of that disease. It is calculated as follows:

Prevalence per 1,000 = [(Number of cases) / (Number of persons in population at the current time)] x 1,000

Diagnostic testing

Assessing validity:

- Sensitivity is defined as the proportion of individuals correctly identified as positive by a particular test. It is expressed as a percent.
- Specificity is defined as the proportion of disease-free individuals identified as negative by a particular diagnostic test. It is also expressed as a percent.
- Positive predictive value is defined as the proportion of individuals who test positive that actually have the disease. It is expressed as a percent.
- Negative predictive value is defined as the proportion of individuals who test negative that are disease-free. It is also expressed as a percent.

Case studies

Case-control studies

In a case-control study, the researcher begins with a group of individuals with the disease of interest (cases) and a comparable disease-free group (controls). The groups are then examined for the history of exposure to the factor of interest. The goal is to determine if a particular factor increases the risk of developing a particular disease.

Cohort studies

In a cohort study, the investigator begins with a group of individuals with a history of exposure to the factor of interest and a comparable group of non-exposed individuals. The groups can then be followed for a period of time to identify the development of a disease (prospective cohort study). An investigator can also begin with a group of individuals whose exposure was documented at a certain time in the past as well as a comparable group of non-exposed people. Records can then be examined to determine the number who developed the disease of interest (retrospective cohort study).

Cross-sectional studies

A cross-sectional study is a study in which exposure to a particular risk factor and development of a disease are assessed simultaneously. This type of study measures prevalent cases of the disease of interest and is also known as a prevalence study. A cross-sectional study cannot assess risk because the chronology of the risk factor and disease development are not known. Cross-sectional studies can only identify an association between a certain factor and disease development and suggest possible risk. The advantages of cross-sectional studies are that they are generally quicker to complete and the cost is lower.

Factors affecting studies

- Confounding occurs when a variable that is a known risk factor for a disease is associated with the factor being studied. An example is a study looking at the relationship between drinking coffee and pancreatic cancer. Smoking is associated with drinking coffee and is known to be a risk factor for pancreatic cancer. Therefore, an observed association between coffee drinking and pancreatic cancer may not be causal, but it may be due to the confounding factor of smoking.
- Recall bias occurs in case-control studies when the cases studied recall issues differently based on their situation. It is also known as rumination bias.

- Selection bias is an error in the selection of the study groups that changes the study outcome. An example of a selection bias occurs when a particular segment of a group being studied is less likely to complete a survey or follow through with the entire study.
- A type I error, or alpha, is the probability that the study will conclude that there is a difference between the intervention group and the control when in fact no difference exists. This is also known as the P-value. The P-value identifies whether or not a result is statistically significant. A $P<0.5$ is considered significant. This means there is less than a five percent chance that no real difference between the two groups exists.
- A type II error, or beta - the study will conclude there is no difference between the groups, when in fact a difference does exist.

Medicare and Medicaid

An individual is eligible for Medicare if they are age 65 years or older and are either receiving or are eligible to receive social security benefits. They are also eligible when not yet 65 years old if they are receiving social security disability benefits or have end-stage renal disease. Part A of Medicare is free and covers inpatient costs, nursing facilities, home health care, and hospice care. Part B requires a premium payment and covers outpatient care, x-rays, and lab work. Part C (Medicare Advantage) covers enrollment in HMOs or PPOs if they are approved. Part D is the Medicare prescription drug benefit. Persons eligible for Medicaid include pregnant women and children under the age of 6 years whose family income is <133% of the poverty level. All children <18 years are eligible if their family income is <100% of the poverty level. Elderly and disabled individuals who are below the poverty level are also eligible.

Obesity

Obesity is defined as being greater than 20% above one's ideal body weight. It is estimated that approximately one third of Americans are obese. Family history, increased age, and female gender all increase the risk of obesity. Obesity is most often caused by a poor diet and sedentary lifestyle. Occasionally, obesity can be due to a medical condition such as hypothyroidism or Cushing's disease, or as it can be a side effect of a medication. Obesity increases an individual's risk of cardiovascular disease, stroke, diabetes, hypertension, and certain cancers. Treatment options include dietary changes, exercise, and other lifestyle changes. Drug therapy can sometimes be helpful. Medications that decrease appetite or reduce fat absorption have been shown to be helpful. In severe cases, weight-loss surgery may be considered. Body mass index is an approximation of body fat based on height and weight. It is calculated by dividing weight (kilograms) by height (in meters squared): BMI = weight (kg) / height (m^2).

Abuse

Child abuse

Child abuse includes the physical, psychological, or sexual mistreatment of a child. Neglect is also a form of child abuse. Child abuse can occur in any socioeconomic or ethnic group. Physicians are mandated to report cases of suspected child abuse. Signs exhibited by children that should arouse suspicion of abuse include a sudden change in behavior, missing school, social withdrawal, and inappropriate sexual behavior. Unexplained cuts, bruises, or burns are also indications there may be abuse. A parental explanation that is vague, changes, or inconsistent with the injuries seen is also a reason to suspect abuse. If abuse is suspected, appropriate authorities must be notified. Careful documentation of the history and injuries is important. Photographs of injuries should be taken.

Domestic violence/partner abuse

Domestic abuse often begins subtly and progresses over time. Initial signs include a partner that is overly controlling and jealous. The abuser is often extremely controlling of finances, social activities, and even everyday issues such as clothing. This can progress to threats, physical and sexual violence. Signs that should lead to suspicion of domestic partner abuse include inconsistent or implausible explanation of injuries, frequent emergency room visits, or delay in seeking medical care. Women are far more likely to be abused by their male partners. Same sex couples are estimated to have about the same incidence of abuse as heterosexual couples. An abused partner is most likely to be killed when attempting to leave the relationship. Mandatory reporting of domestic violence is not required in most states.

Elder abuse

The different types of elder abuse include physical, sexual, emotional, financial, and neglect. The most likely perpetrator is a family member. Institutional caregivers are also potential abusers of the elderly. Women and individuals over the age of 80 years are more likely to be abused. The more dependent an elderly individual, the greater the chances of abuse. Signs of abuse include unexplained cuts, bruises, burns, or other injuries. Weight loss, poor hygiene, and other unmet needs are also signs that there may be abuse. Improper management of valuables and finances should also lead to suspicion of abuse. Physicians should routinely question elderly patients about the possibility of abuse and take appropriate action if abuse is suspected.

AMA code of medical ethics

The AMA code of medical ethics is a set of standards developed by the American Medical Association that physicians are expected to adhere. The code of medical ethics was first developed and published in 1847. It is revised on a regular basis. There are nine basic principles that make up the code. In summary, the nine principles state that a physician should: be dedicated and competent and uphold standards of professionalism at all times. Physicians should abide by the law and respect the rights and privacy of patients. A physician should commit to continuing medical education and to improving the health of the community. The principles also state that physicians are free to choose where and to whom they will provide medical care, except in cases of an emergency.

Herbal medicines

There are numerous herbal medicines are readily available over the counter for patients. Most are safe, but some can have toxic effects or unwanted drug interactions. Some of the more commonly used herbal remedies include aloe vera gel for burn relief, Echinacea for colds and flu, ginseng for numerous disorders, and green tea extract as an antioxidative medication. Some common herbal remedies with potentially toxic effects include kava (which is toxic to the liver and may alter the effect of other medications), ephedra (which can cause palpitations and other autonomic hyperactivity), and ginseng (which may be linked to some unwanted health effects). Patients should routinely be asked about their use of herbal remedies and advised accordingly.

Psychiatry

Dysthymia

Dysthymia is defined as mood disorder characterized by episodes of mild to moderate depression. Symptoms are similar to those of a major depression, but less severe. It is very common and can affect all age groups. Presenting symptoms include fatigue, poor appetite, difficulty sleeping and concentrating, loss of interest in daily activities, and a feeling of hopelessness. In order to fulfill the DSM-5 criteria, patients must have at least two of the symptoms on most days for at least two years. Patients cannot have a symptom-free period of longer than two months and symptoms must interfere with their daily activities. There must not be evidence for any other disorder causing the symptoms. Treatment includes psychotherapy and antidepressant medication.

Major depressive disorder

Major depressive disorder is a severe depression that has a significant impact on the ability of an individual to carry out their daily activities. To fulfill the DSM-5 criteria, a patient must have at least five of the following symptoms for at least a two week period: depressed mood lasting most of the day, decreased interest in normal daily activities, weight gain or loss, sleep disturbance, lack of energy, feelings of worthlessness or helplessness, difficulty concentrating, suicidal ideation. The cause of depression is unknown. It can be diagnosed at any age and women are affected more frequently than men. There is an increased risk in individuals with a family history of major depression. Treatment options include antidepressant medication, psychotherapy, and electroconvulsive therapy (ECT). Complications include suicide, alcohol and substance abuse, work and social problems.

Postpartum major depression

Postpartum major depression is defined as a significant episode of depression occurring in the postpartum period. It is extremely common in up to 10% of postpartum women. The onset can be anywhere from one day to several months post delivery. Postpartum major depression must be distinguished from "baby blues", which is a mild transient form of postpartum depression that generally begins about 4 days following delivery and resolves by day 10. The diagnosis is generally made clinically after a thorough psychiatric evaluation. Treatment options include counseling and antidepressant medications. Selective serotonin reuptake inhibitors (SSRIs) and tricyclic antidepressants (TCAs) can be used; however, they are excreted into the breast milk, and therefore caution should be used with breast-feeding mothers. Complications include postpartum psychosis. This affects approximately 0.2% of postpartum women. Postpartum psychosis increases the risk of the mother harming herself or her baby and is a psychiatric emergency.

Bipolar disorders

Bipolar disorder is a mood disorder characterized by separate episodes of both mania and depression. There are two forms of the disease. In bipolar I disorder, there must be a history of at least one manic episode. In bipolar II disorder, a patient has recurrent depressive episodes along with hypomanic, not manic, episodes. To qualify as a manic episode, symptoms must last a minimum of four days and lead to difficulties with work or social life. Hypomanic episodes must last a minimum of four days, but do not cause work or social problems.

Diagnosis and treatment

Bipolar disorder is estimated to affect 1% of the population. Men and women are equally affected. The average age of onset is between the ages of 15 to 30 years. Patients present with a history of alternating episodes of mania and depression. Manic symptoms include feelings of euphoria, poor judgment, risk behavior, inappropriate spending, and hypersexuality. Symptoms of depression include feelings of sadness or hopelessness, sleep or appetite disturbance, loss of interest in activities, and suicidal ideation. Treatment options include mood stabilizers such as lithium. Antidepressants may trigger manic episodes and are not usually recommended. Complications include suicide, alcohol and substance abuse, financial, work and social problems.

Premenstrual syndrome

Premenstrual syndrome refers to a group of physical and psychological symptoms that occur in relation to a woman's menstrual cycle. Premenstrual dysphoric disorder is a severe form of premenstrual syndrome. It is estimated that up to 80% of women experience some symptoms of premenstrual syndrome. Approximately 3 to 5% of women are diagnosed with premenstrual dysphoric disorder. Symptoms include anxiety, depression, mood swings, bloating and weight gain, headaches, and joint pains occurring in the mid-luteal phase of the menstrual cycle. The diagnosis is made based on the history. Treatments include lifestyle and dietary changes such as decreasing caffeine and sodium intake. Nutritional supplementation includes the use of vitamin B_6, vitamin E, calcium, magnesium, and tryptophan. Antidepressants are sometimes used for severe symptoms. Oral contraceptives and Depo-Provera® have also been used to treat premenstrual dysphoric disorder.

Generalized anxiety disorder

Generalized anxiety disorder is defined as excessive and disproportionate worry and anxiety lasting a minimum of six months. The disorder generally has its onset in childhood, adolescence, or as a young adult and is more common in girls. It tends to be chronic and recurrent. Patients complain of feeling stressed and worried. Patients also complain of difficulty concentrating or sleeping. The diagnosis is made clinically after ruling out medical causes such as thyroid disease. Treatments include benzodiazepines, antidepressants, and cognitive behavioral therapy.

Panic disorder

Panic disorder is characterized by the occurrence of sudden, unexpected episodes of intense anxiety. Patients complain of sudden onset of tachycardia, shortness of breath, sweating, choking sensation, and a feeling of imminent death. Panic attacks generally last from several minutes to an hour. Complications include difficulties with work, school, or social situations. At times, patients develop phobias (e.g., school phobia). Treatment options include SSRIs, benzodiazepines, and cognitive behavioral therapy.

Obsessive-compulsive disorder

Obsessive-compulsive disorder (OCD) is a psychiatric disorder characterized by recurrence of unwanted, distressing thoughts or the need to repeatedly perform certain behaviors or rituals. Obsessive-compulsive disorder is common and usually has its onset in childhood or adolescence. Patients present with a history of obsessive thoughts. These include obsessive fears about things like dirt or being contaminated or fears that they have hurt someone or are going to hurt someone. Patients may also exhibit compulsive behaviors like repeated hand washing, counting, or arranging of items. The diagnosis of obsessive-compulsive disorder can be made if the patient realizes that the obsessions or compulsions are not reasonable and that they interfere with daily activities. Treatment options include cognitive behavioral therapy and antidepressants.

Review Video: Obsessive-Compulsive Disorder (OCD)
Visit mometrix.com/academy and enter code: 499790

Schizophrenia

Schizophrenia is a chronic psychiatric disorder characterized by an impaired perception of reality. Schizophrenia is common, affecting approximately 1% of the population. Men and women are equally affected; however, men are typically diagnosed in their late teens and twenties and women are usually diagnosed in their late twenties to forties. Men tend to have a more severe disease. Having a family history of schizophrenia increases the risk of developing the condition. Patients usually present with delusions and hallucinations. Patients can exhibit inappropriate speech, outbursts, and bizarre behavior. The severity of symptoms varies considerably. The diagnosis requires that patients must have at least two symptoms for a minimum of six months. Symptoms must disrupt their daily activities. Medical causes must be ruled out. Treatment is with antipsychotic medications. The new generation antipsychotics are preferred because they do not cause tardive dyskinesia. Psychotherapy is also used.

Personality disorders

Personality disorders are defined by the American Psychiatric Association as, "an enduring pattern of inner experience and behavior that deviates markedly from the expectations of the culture of the individual who exhibits it." Personality disorders are divided into three clusters. Cluster A refers to the odd or eccentric personality disorders. They include paranoid, schizoid, and schizotypal personality disorders. Cluster B contains the emotional personality disorders such antisocial, borderline, histrionic, and narcissistic. Cluster C includes the anxious or fearful personality disorders such as avoidant, dependent, or obsessive-compulsive. Presenting symptoms depend on the specific personality disorder. Complications can include substance abuse, social isolation, depression, and suicide. Treatment is generally psychotherapy. Medications are of limited use.

Practice Test

1. A 16-year-old boy presents with right shoulder pain after being hit during a neighborhood football game while he was attempting to throw the ball. He resists any arm motion and cradles it. During examination, dimpling is noted inferior to the acromion. What is the most likely diagnosis?

a. Rotator cuff tear
b. Shoulder dislocation
c. Rotator cuff impingement
d. Rupture of the long head of the biceps

2. A 42-year-old woman experiences progressively increasing right foot pain that developed during her regular running routine. She states that at first, she would get relief from resting and icing her foot, but now that no longer helps. She now notes midfoot pain even at night and has had to stop running. What is the most likely diagnosis?

a. Tendonitis
b. Plantar fasciitis
c. Metatarsal stress fracture
d. Jones fracture

3. Patients with low back pain should be referred to a specialist if they experience

a. chronic sciatica for 6 or more weeks or new or progressive neurologic deficit.
b. herniated nucleus pulposus (HNP) with major muscle weakness.
d. recurrent back pain.
d. A and B only.
e. all of the above.

4. In pharmacologic treatment of patients with mechanical low back pain (LBP), which of the following is true?

a. Acetaminophen is one of the best first line treatments, followed by NSAIDs.
b. NSAIDs and muscle relaxants work better when in conjunction with one another.
c. Opioids are a typical first-line treatment.
d. A and B are true.
e. All of the above are true.

5. A patient presents with a whiplash injury. Upon examination, the patient experiences paraesthesias along the spine when the neck is flexed. This is a positive

a. Lhermitte sign.
b. Lachman test.
c. Spurling test.
d. blocker, beggar, kisser, grabber, Spock sign.

6. A 46-year-old Caucasian woman with a family history of basal cell carcinoma but no melanomas presents to a clinic with concerns regarding skin cancer. She has numerous nevi, freckles, and some atypical looking nevi. On examination, the physician notes 2 asymmetric nevi with irregular borders. What is the best way to counsel her?

a. Tell her that recent studies show that due to her family history, she has an 80% lifetime risk of developing malignant melanoma.
b. Counsel her that she has no need to see a dermatologist for a risk assessment.
c. Be watchful for nevi with malignant features and counsel her regarding self-examination.
d. Tell her the best approach to the biopsy of the suspicious nevi is a shave biopsy.

7. An 8-month-old boy presents with several large crusted, scaly lesions on his face and a few on the extensor surface of his arms. His mother notes that the lesions bother him, and he tends to scratch at them. According to the mother the lesions have been present for approximately 1 month and appear to be spreading. What is the most likely diagnosis?

a. Atopic dermatitis
b. Psoriasis
c. Seborrheic dermatitis
d. Tinea corporis

8. A 17-year-old girl presents with moderate acne including papules, pustules, and a few nodules. She has been using over-the-counter benzoyl peroxide, which is no longer helping. What is the best line of treatment?

a. Isotretinoin
b. Topical erythromycin 3% + 5% benzoyl peroxide
c. 5% benzoyl peroxide
d. Oral once-daily minocycline

9. During a routine well examination, a 62-year-old man is found to have Hgb of 11.5 g/dL. He admits to a poor diet. Further laboratory work reveals hypersegmented neutrophils, MCV of 120 fL, total serum iron of 155, vitamin B_{12} of 176 pg/mL, RBC folate of 130 pg/L, and a reticulocyte count of 1.1%. This patient has

a. anemia of chronic disease.
b. vitamin B12 deficiency.
c. iron deficiency anemia.
d. folic acid deficiency.

10. A patient, who is on day 5 of penicillin for strep pharyngitis, complains of increased headaches, exhaustion, and jaundice. Laboratory work reveals Hgb 9.2 g/dL, increased indirect bilirubin, a low serum haptoglobin level, and a positive direct Coombs test. This patient most likely has

a. mononucleosis.
b. autoimmune hemolytic anemia.
c. hereditary spherocytosis.
d. resistant streptococcal pharyngitis.

11. What is the best way to treat hypertension in a patient with stage 3 chronic kidney disease?

a. Advise the patient to decrease their protein, sodium, and alcohol intake to control their hypertension.
b. Use calcium channel blockers and β-blockers in combination.
c. Use angiotensin-converting enzyme inhibitors (ACEI), angiotensin II receptor blockers (ARB), and loop diuretics in combination.
d. Use diuretics, as they are the best treatment at this stage.

12. A 33-year-old man presents with pain on urination, increasing back pain, and fever. He states that he avoided coming in for examination until he could no longer tolerate the pain, which is now sharp and stabbing. He also states that he has been having difficulty urinating. On examination there is pronounced left flank pain and a palpable left kidney. Urine dipstick reveals positive nitrites and hematuria. The physician suspects and must immediately rule out which of the following conditions?

a. Pyonephrosis
b. Pyelonephritis complicated with nephrolithiasis
c. Pyelonephritis and dehydration
d. Staghorn calculus

13. A patient presents with acute right upper quadrant (RUQ) pain. What imaging study is the test of choice to assess this patient?

a. Ultrasound (US)
b. Plain films
c. Abdominal computed tomography (CT)
d. Endoscopy

14. A 74-year-old woman reports that she has experienced "crampy" left lower quadrant abdominal pain with diarrhea for 4 days. On examination, she has a temperature of 101.5 °F, pulse of 110 beats per minute, decreased capillary refill, and moderate left lower quadrant abdominal pain. The complete blood count shows leukocytosis with a left shift. An abdominal CT helps diagnose diverticulitis and rules out an abscess. What is the best course of treatment?

a. Instruct the patient to follow a clear liquid diet and return to the office in 2 days for a follow-up appointment.
b. Instruct the patient to follow a clear liquid diet with ciprofloxacin and metronidazole for 10 days.
c. Instruct the patient to follow a clear liquid diet with ciprofloxacin and metronidazole for 10 days, plus add ibuprofen for the pain.
d. Hospitalize the patient with complete bowel rest and broad-spectrum intravenous antibiotics.

15. A 55 year-old-woman, who was previously diagnosed with irritable bowel syndrome (IBS) at another office, presents with complaints of dyspepsia, diarrhea, bloating, and weight loss. She has been following a high-fiber diet, including many whole-grain breads, and avoiding dairy and other fatty foods. She is frustrated as her symptoms have not improved and seem to be getting worse. Due to the patient's history, the physician should suspect which of the following?

a. Worsening IBS
b. Viral gastroenteritis
c. Ulcerative colitis
d. Celiac disease

16. The physician orders an electrocardiograph (ECG) of a 44-year-old patient with hypertension. The ECG shows left ventricular hypertrophy (LVH). Which of these findings should the physician expect to see in this ECG?

a. A tall R wave in V6, a deep S in V1, inverted T waves in V5 and V6, and left axis deviation
b. A predominant R wave in V1, a deep S in V6, inverted T waves in V2 and V3, and right axis deviation
c. A tall R wave in V6, a deep S in V1, inverted T waves in V5 and V6, and right axis deviation
d. A predominant R wave in V1, a deep S in V6, inverted T waves in V2 and V3, and left axis deviation

17. Which statement is FALSE regarding B-type natriuretic peptide (BNP)?

a. It is a cardiac neurohormone that is secreted from the ventricles due to volume expansion and pressure overload.
b. Levels increase in patients with CHF and vary in proportion to the exacerbation of the overload.
c. Levels greater than 400 pg/mL indicate a definitive diagnosis of congestive heart failure (CHF) and are good to screen for and monitor CHF.
d. BNP levels are lower in men than women, are inversely related to body weight, and increase with age.

18. According to the ACC/AHA (American College of Cardiology/American Heart Association), when should one add β-blockers to a patient with Stage B heart failure (HF) who is already being treated with an ACE inhibitor (angiotensin converting enzyme) or ARB (angiotensin receptor blocker)?

a. Only in a patient with a previous MI (myocardial infarction), regardless of ejection fraction (EF)
b. In a patient with a decreased EF and a history of more than 1 MI
c. In a patient with a recent MI, regardless of EF, or a decreased EF regardless of history of MI
d. None of the above (β-blockers are not used until Stage C)

19. A 46-year-old man's fasting lipid profile shows a total cholesterol of 238 mg/dL, HDL-C (high-density lipoprotein cholesterol) of 41 mg/dL, and a LDL-C (low-density lipoprotein cholesterol) of 185. He has a 100 pack-year history of smoking. According to the Framingham Coronary Risk Calculator, he is in the moderately high risk category (10-year risk = 10-20%). The goal for this patient's LDL cholesterol is less than

a. 70 mg/dL.
b. 130 mg/dL.
c. 100 mg/dL.
d. 160 mg/dL.

20. In the above patient (Question #19), who has a blood pressure (BP) of 129/82, which first line of pharmacotherapy for hyperlipidemia would be best?

a. Lovastatin
b. Nicotinic acid
c. Ezetimibe
d. Niacin

21. Which statement is true regarding atrial fibrillation (AF)?

a. 20% of new patients spontaneously convert to a normal sinus rhythm in 48 hours.
b. When treating AF, quality of life is increased with rhythm control over rate control.
c. There is no difference in quality of life between rhythm and rate control in patients with AF.
d. Use the 1,2,3 Cardioversion Rule when approaching patients with AF in regard to duration and anticoagulation use.

22. A 36-year-old woman presents during a screening thyroid stimulating hormone (TSH) test with a TSH of 12 μIU/mL. Further testing shows a normal Free T3 and Free T4. What is true of this patient?

a. She has subclinical hypothyroidism with a high risk of developing true hypothyroidism.
b. She has subclinical hypothyroidism with a low risk of developing true hypothyroidism.
c. She has primary hypothyroidism.
d. She has Hashimoto thyroiditis.

23. A 27-year-old woman complains of difficulty conceiving. She notes sudden weight gain, irregular menstrual cycles, acne, and hirsutism. The physician should suspect which of the following conditions?

a. Graves disease
b. Addison's disease
c. Hyperparathyroidism
d. Cushing syndrome

24. When a 34-year-old diabetic patient comes in for a diabetic follow-up, the physician discovers that she is pregnant with her first child. She is doing well on metformin and her B_{12} is normal, but she has questions regarding its safety in pregnancy. The physician should advise her of which of the following?

a. Metformin is safe in pregnancy and she won't have to monitor her B12 while pregnant.
b. She may use it while pregnant, but will have to change medications if she plans to breastfeed.
c. She will need to change diabetic medications since metformin is category C in pregnancy.
d. None of the above is true.

25. Parkinson's is diagnosed based on the presence of which of the following symptoms?

a. Hyperkinesia, resting tremor, muscular rigidity, and postural instability
b. Bradykinesia, intentional tremor, muscular instability, and dyskinesia
c. Hyperkinesia, resting tremor, myoclonus, and dyskinesia
d. Bradykinesia, resting tremor, muscular rigidity, and postural instability

26. A complex partial seizure includes which of the following symptoms?

a. Impaired consciousness and altered behavior or repetitive motions
b. Retained consciousness, altered behavior, and an aura
c. Retained consciousness, a blank stare, and generalized jerking
d. Impaired consciousness, an aura, and the Jacksonian march

27. When treating influenza, one must be aware of which of the following?

a. Influenza A includes H1N1 and H3N2, which can be treated with antivirals.
b. Treatment must be started within 48 hours or it won't benefit the patient at all.
c. Both oseltamivir and zanamivir are effective against both influenza type A and B.
d. Both A and C are true.
e. All of the above are true.

28. Which is true regarding acute bronchitis?

a. Antibiotics should be used if the cough is present for more than 2 weeks in all patients, regardless of age.
b. Antibiotics should be used if elderly (older than 65) and if the patient was hospitalized in the last year, has diabetes, congestive heart failure, or is on steroids.
c. Patients with an acute exacerbation of chronic bronchitis should not be treated with antibiotics.
d. Bronchodilators should be reserved for those who are on antibiotics.

29. A previously healthy 66-year-old patient presents with a 5-day history of a productive cough, temperature of 101.8 °F, BP of 110/75, pulse of 95 beats/min, and a respiratory rate of 21/min. On examination, the physician finds the patient to be alert and oriented with rales in the right lower lobe. Laboratory tests indicate an elevated white count and BUN of 18. A chest x-ray confirms right lower lobe pneumonia. Which of the following is true?

a. According to CURB-65, this patient has a score of 3 and will respond best to IV antibiotics and must be hospitalized.
b. The gold standard to diagnose pneumonia is the detection of rales or crackles on examination.
c. According to CURB-65, this patient has a score of 1 and may be treated as an outpatient for community acquired pneumonia.
d. Community-acquired pneumonia should only be treated with combination antibiotic therapy.

30. Which is true regarding step 3 (moderate/persistent) asthma in patients age 6 to adults?

a. Symptoms occur less than twice a week, exacerbations may affect daily activities, and nighttime symptoms occur more than 2 times per month.
b. Exacerbations occur frequently and asthma symptoms are continual with frequent nighttime episodes.
c. Exacerbations are brief and of varying intensities and nighttime symptoms occur twice a month or less.
d. Symptoms occur daily with exacerbations at least twice a week which may last for several days, while nighttime symptoms occur more than once per week.

31. In the above patient (Question #30), which is the best treatment?

a. Daily medication should include a leukotriene modifier, theophylline, or low-dose inhaled corticosteroid.
b. No daily medication is required, only a short-acting β2 agonist as needed.
c. Daily medications include either a low or medium-dose inhaled corticosteroid plus a long-acting bronchodilator.
d. Daily medications include a high-dose inhaled corticosteroid, a long-acting bronchodilator, an oral corticosteroid, and a leukotriene modifier.
e. None of the above is the best treatment.

32. Which is true regarding COPD (chronic obstructive pulmonary disease)?

a. Spirometry remains the mainstay for diagnosing COPD, with a FEV1/FVC (forced expiratory volume in 1 second over forced vital capacity) of less than 70% of predicted being diagnostic.
b. Symptoms usually occur when the percent predicted postbronchodilator FEV1 falls below 80%.
c. Arterial blood gases provide the best clues to the length and severity of an exacerbation.
d. All of the above are true.

33. A 19-year-old man presents with a 1-day history of increasing right-sided testicular pain and swelling. The patient is afebrile and experiencing nausea without vomiting. The physician must rule out which disease process since it is a true surgical emergency?

a. Orchitis
b. Testicular torsion
c. Epididymitis
d. Spermatocele

34. Dysmenorrhea is the most common gynecologic complaint among women of child-bearing years, and it is important to distinguish between primary and secondary dysmenorrhea. Which of the following is true regarding dysmenorrhea?

a. In patients presenting with complaints of painful menses, one should perform a pelvic examination with cervical smear and cultures only if one suspects secondary dysmenorrhea.
b. Primary dysmenorrhea typically begins within the first 6 months of menarche, patients note pain beginning with the onset of menstruation which lasts 12-72 hours, and the pain responds well to prostaglandin inhibitors.
c. Diagnostic laparoscopy is required for a definitive diagnosis.
d. Secondary dysmenorrhea involves underlying pelvic disease, typically appears in one's 20s or 30s and responds very well to oral contraceptives (OCs) or NSAIDs.

35. In patients with abnormal uterine bleeding, who should receive an endometrial biopsy?

a. Women over 30
b. Women with chronic ovulation
c. Women with prolonged periods of unopposed estrogen
d. Underweight women

36. The differential diagnosis for acute gynecologic causes for abdominal pain in non-pregnant patients includes all of the following EXCEPT

a. pelvic inflammatory disease (PID).
b. endometriosis.
c. uterine leiomyomas.
d. ruptured ovarian cyst.

37. When treating depression in the elderly, which of the following should be avoided due to its potential for cardiotoxic side effects?

a. Fluoxetine
b. Amitriptyline
c. Bupropion
d. Venlafaxine

38. A 29-year-old man presents with complaints of difficulty sleeping, difficulty concentrating, and increased irritability. He admits that he feels tense most of the time and that these symptoms have increased over the last 8 months after his company downsized. He fears that he will lose his job due to his increasing inability to focus. These symptoms are increasingly affecting his home life and other relationships. This patient most likely has which of the following conditions?

a. Generalized anxiety disorder
b. Panic disorder
c. Social phobia
d. Specific phobia

39. Somatoform disorders may be distinguished from malingering by which of the following?

a. Somatoform disorders may be linked to an underlying medical condition while malingering may not.
b. Symptoms are willfully produced in somatoform disorders in order to seek attention while they are not willful in malingering patients.
c. Malingering presents with multiple episodes of different problems while somatoform disorders presents with multiple episodes of the same problem.
d. Neither may be linked to an underlying medical condition and in somatoform disorders symptoms are not willful while they are willfully produced in malingering.

40. A new couple brings in their 4-year-old child for a well-child check. You discover that their primary source of water is from a well and test for fluoride. Tests results show 0.4 ppm (parts per million). The physician should advise the parents of which of the following?

a. No fluoride treatment is necessary until the child reaches adolescence.
b. No fluoride treatment is necessary unless the child is less than 1 year old.
c. Fluoride supplements should be provided through 16 years old.
d. Fluoride should be provided until the child is 6 years old.

41. Which treatment for acute otitis media (AOM) is best in a 14 month old with bilateral AOM, fever, ear pain, and no antibiotic use in the last 30 days?

a. Withhold treatment for 48-72 hours to see if the patient spontaneously resolves.
b. After treating with antibiotics, start prophylactic antibiotics for 3 months since the patient is less than 18 months old.
c. Begin amoxicillin at 80-90 mg/kg/day.
d. Recommend NSAIDs for pain and reevaluate the child within 48 hours.

42. Which is true regarding travelers' diarrhea?

a. It is usually self-limiting within 5-7 days
b. Trimethoprim-sulfamethoxazole or doxycycline is the treatment of choice.
c. There is increasing resistance of Campylobacter infections to azithromycin.
d. Ciprofloxacin is the drug of choice unless pregnant or a child, then, azithromycin should be prescribed.

43. Which of the following FALSE regarding presbycusis?

a. Presbycusis is a bilateral high-frequency sensorineural hearing loss that increases with age.
b. Presbycusis can lead to depression and sense of isolation since it causes difficulty is speech discrimination.
c. Patients typically seek help early on in the disease process.
d. The whisper test is abnormal as the level of hearing loss increases; however, the Weber and Rinne test remain normal.

44. Which of the following is not a risk factor for cataracts?

a. Poor diet and insufficient vitamin intake
b. Ultraviolet light exposure
c. Glaucoma
d. Smoking and alcohol use

45. In July 2013, the American Academy of Otolaryngology-Head and Neck Surgery Foundation (AAO-HNSF) issued an evidence-based guideline for tympanostomy tube use in children 6 months to 12 years old with otitis media (OM). Which of the following is true?

a. Tympanostomy tubes should be placed if bilateral OME (otitis media with effusion) persists for more than 3 months with the presence of hearing impairment.
b. Tympanostomy tubes should be placed if unilateral OME persists for 2 months.
c. Children with tympanostomy tubes who develop OM should be placed on oral and topical antibiotics.
d. Children with tympanostomy tubes should always wear earplugs when swimming or bathing.

46. Preventative services for the elderly should include all of the following EXCEPT

a. annual influenza vaccine, one time zoster vaccine, and a one-time pneumococcal vaccine for those older than 65 years.
b. colon cancer screening up to 75 years old and breast cancer screening every 2 years up to 74 years old.
c. aspirin therapy in men 45-79 and women 55-79 years old when the benefits outweigh the GI (gastrointestinal) bleeding risk.
d. annual abdominal aortic aneurism in men 65-75 years old.

47. When facing issues surrounding a patient and genetic testing, one should consider which of the following legal issues?

a. Privacy and confidentiality
b. Insurance and employment discrimination
c. Informed consent
d. Duty to warn at-risk-relatives if they are in clear and imminent danger
e. All of the above

48. Focusing on a good therapeutic alliance between the patient and physician in the primary care setting involves all of the following EXCEPT

a. establishing a good bond between the physician and patient through good communication.
b. the physician relying on thorough medical knowledge alone.
c. respectful and nonjudgmental communication increases good health care by enlisting the trust of the patient, and so improves the patient's adherence to treatment.
d. the ability of the physician to translate medical information to the patient.

49. Culturally competent medical care helps to ensure quality medical care by recognizing that culture shapes the way patients interprets which of the following?

a. How diseases are classified and what causes disease
b. Relationship between the healer, sick person, and their family
c. How the body functions normally
d. How they select a healer
e. All of the above

50. The mainstay of palliative medicine is pain control. Which of the following is FALSE regarding the general use of opioids and pain medications in palliative or hospice care?

a. Chronic pain needs around-the-clock medication.
b. Codeine is the most commonly used opioid.
c. Breakthrough pain should receive prn (as needed) medication at 10-15% of the 24-hour dose.
d. Parenteral opioids are preferred when pain is severe due to their quick onset of action and ease of titration.

Answer Key and Explanations

1. B: Patients with rotator cuff tears can present with pain stiffness and occasional weakness around the shoulder, but are often asymptomatic. The symptoms typically have an insidious onset. With a complete tear, patients often exhibit a "drop arm sign" where the arm drops with abduction. Shoulder dislocations are typically sports-related in younger patients and the result of a fall in the elderly. Patients resist or refuse to move their arm. They usually occur when the injury involves the arm in abduction and maximal external rotation. The humeral head can typically be visualized as a bulge and dimpling occurs just inferior to the acromion where the humeral head should be. Rotator cuff impingement is a mainly a clinical diagnosis. The patient presents with dull shoulder pain increasing over weeks to months. The pain is exacerbated during the night with various sleeping positions, especially when the arm is overhead. Range of motion (ROM) is usually normal. However, a painful arc of motion may be noted especially on internal rotation and forward flexion. The "empty can test" (thumb pointing downward with arm abducted 90° and with 30° forward flexion) can test for supraspinatus strength. Finally, patients with a rupture of the long head of the biceps usually present with a rotator cuff tear. With the rupture, the patient notes a pop followed by an immediate decrease in symptoms. Physical examination reveals anterior bruising and a "Popeye muscle" upon flexion of the biceps.

2. C: Tendonitis would elicit specific pain along the offending tendon and is typically described as an acute burning or stabbing pain. Plantar fasciitis is common in runners, and is worse in the morning or after prolonged periods of rest when standing. The pain is located on the plantar surface of the heel, usually with pain upon palpation along the anteromedial section of the calcaneus. Metatarsal stress fractures or "March fractures" are very common in athletes and have an insidious onset. It typically involves the 2nd metatarsal followed by the 3rd and 4th due to the amount of weight-bearing load. Therefore midfoot or forefoot pain is most commonly described by the patient. While Jones fractures are also metatarsal fractures, they are acute and involve the proximal 5th metatarsal.

3. E: Low back pain (LBP) is the second most common condition encountered in primary care only after upper respiratory infections. This is a significant health problem that can lead to chronic disability. Because of this, it is important to recognize red flags and to determine when a patient should be referred. Red flags include evidence for cancer, infection, acute abdominal aneurysm, fracture, cauda equina syndrome, history of trauma, and neurologic deficit. In the absence of abnormal findings on examination/radiography/laboratory work, and after patients have been treated conservatively for 4-6 weeks, they should be referred to a program that will help them return to normal function especially if it's recurrent or chronic. Patients should be referred to a rheumatologist when inflammatory arthropathy, fibromyalgia, or metabolic bone disease are suspected. Neurology referrals are appropriate when there is sciatica for more than 6 weeks, a new or progressive motor deficit is present, or the patient has leg pain with a negative straight-leg-raise test. Neurosurgery consults are necessary when the herniated disk (HNP) is significant and associated with major muscle weakness.

4. D: LBP may be classified as nonspecific or mechanical, LBP possibly caused by radiculopathy or spinal stenosis, or LBP with possible other causes due to presence of red flags. When it is determined that LBP is mechanical (or nonspecific and lasting less than 4weeks), pharmacotherapy may include acetaminophen, NSAIDs, muscle relaxants, or opioids. Acetaminophen remains one of the best first-line treatments because of its efficacy and low side-effect profile. Studies suggest that NSAIDs and muscle relaxants work better when used concurrently and are frequently prescribed together in the primary care setting. Opioids are reserved for extreme pain since they are only

slightly more effective than other analgesics and can lead to dependency. Topically applied lidocaine patches are also useful in acute LBP.

5. A: The Lhermitte sign is positive for when the patient experiences paraesthesias along the spine or upper extremities when the head flexes anteriorly. This may indicate spondylosis, multiple sclerosis, or myelopathy. The Lachman test checks for anterior cruciate ligament injury in the knee and is characterized by being able to displace the tibia anteriorly. A positive Spurling test involves pain radiating to the posterior shoulder or arm on the ipsilateral downward pressure on the head. This test has a high specificity for cervical radiculopathy. The Blocker (C5), beggar (C6), kisser (C7), grabber (C8), Spock (T1) mnemonic is helpful in remembering the motor innervations of the cervical roots.

6. C: To date no study has documented a way to predict that this patient has an 80% lifetime risk of having melanoma. Risk factors for developing malignant melanoma include changing moles, having dysplastic nevi with a family history of melanoma, having more than 50 nevi (bigger than 2 mm), and having one or more family members with malignant melanoma. Minor risk factors include freckling, sun sensitivity, and a history of severe, blistering sunburns. In the United States the risk for developing malignant melanoma is ~0.6% or 1 in 150. The lifetime risk does increase in familial atypical mole and melanoma syndrome (FAMM). Criteria for FAMM include malignant melanoma in at least one 1st- or 2nd-degree relative, more than 50 nevi (some being atypical), and certain histological changes. This patient does not appear to have FAMM, but does have some risk factors for skin cancer. Due to her risk factors she would benefit from a dermatology consultation. The best way to counsel this patient would be to educate her regarding recognizing the ABC's melanoma as well as being observant. Also, suspicious nevi should have an excisional or punch biopsy.

7. A: Atopic dermatitis typically appears in the first year of life with pruritus being the hallmark of the disease. Lesions usually involve the face in infants become excoriated with weeping and crusting. Eventually lesions become scaly and lichenified. Unlike seborrheic dermatitis, it does not typically follow the distribution of oil glands. Psoriasis typically appears after infancy and tinea corporis spreads slower.

8. B: For moderate acne, topical antibiotics are the treatment of choice and work best in conjunction with benzoyl peroxide. Isotretinoin is reserved for severe nodulocystic acne.

9. D: This patient presents with a macrocytic anemia (nl MCV=80-100 fL and nl male Hgb=13.5-17.5 g/dL). Iron deficiency anemia and anemia of chronic disease are both microcytic anemias. Since the levels of vitamin B_{12}, iron, and reticulocyte count are normal (nl B_{12}=150-900 pg/mL and nl iron=50-170 μg/dL, and nl retic=0.5-1.5%) and folate levels are low (less than 150 pg/L), he must have a folic acid deficiency.

10. B: Penicillin, methyldopa, and quinidine are known to produce a warm antibody autoimmune reaction which is supported by the positive direct Coombs test (indicates hemolysis), elevated indirect bilirubin (increases in hemolysis), and low serum haptoglobin (which indicates a moderate to severe hemolysis).

11. C: Stage 3 of chronic kidney disease is defined as those with a moderate decreased in glomerular filtration rate (GFR) of 30-59. The goal in these patients is to slow the deterioration in renal function, to keep the BP below 130/80 and to protect against cardiovascular disease. The combination of ACEIs, ARBs, and loop diuretics has been shown in multiple trials to help patients protect kidney function while treating hypertension. Although dietary changes are very important, they are not enough to maintain renal function in these patients.

12. A: The patient's initial symptoms are classic for pyelonephritis complicated with nephrolithiasis. However, with the addition of urinary obstruction symptoms, one must rule out the cause of the obstruction. Of the choices for the possible cause of obstruction with an infection (nephrolithiasis and pyonephrosis), pyonephrosis is a true urologic emergency that must be ruled out.

13. A: The American College of Radiology has recommended different imaging studies based on pain location. US is recommended to assess RUQ pain while CT with contrast is best for right lower and left lower quadrant pain (RLQ and LLQ). CT without contrast is recommended for left upper quadrant (LUQ) pain.

14. D: Answer B is the best choice for those with mild diverticulitis who can tolerate oral rehydration. Ibuprofen should not be used in patients with diverticulitis due to the increased risk of GI bleeding. However, this patient exhibits signs of inflammation including fever and leukocytosis and signs of dehydration which require hospitalization. Diverticulitis tends to be more severe in elderly patients.

15. D: The symptoms of IBS and celiac sprue or celiac disease often overlap. These symptoms include diarrhea, flatulence, and abdominal discomfort. The key to this patient was her history of increased ingestion of whole-grain breads, which led to an increase in her symptoms. Ulcerative colitis is marked by bloody diarrhea. IBS is a diagnosis of exclusion and the history did not indicate an acute viral illness.

16. A: Answer A corresponds to changes seen in LVH while answer B corresponds to changes seen in right ventricular hypertrophy. Leads I, aVL, and V4-6 are left-sided leads while leads III, aVR, and V1-3 are right-sided leads. In LVH the ventricular wall is thickened, which results in an increased R wave in the left-sided leads and a deeper S wave in the right-sided leads. Inverted T waves in V5 and V6 show the strain on the left ventricle.

17. C: While a BNP value greater than 400 pg/mL does point to a probable diagnosis of CHF, it is not a definitive diagnosis. One must also rely on the history, physical examination, and other tests. It is not a good test for screening or monitoring since the value changes rapidly in response to volume and pressure overload. However, it is helpful when distinguishing between cardiac and pulmonary causes of dyspnea.

18. C: Once a patient reaches stage B of heart failure, a β-blocker should be added when either of the above situations in answer C is present.

19. B: The goal for a patient's LDL cholesterol is under 100 mg/dL (under 70 is optimal) for high risk, under 130 mg/dL (under 100 optimal) for moderately high risk, under 130 mg/dL for moderate risk, and under 160 mg/dL for patients with 0 to 1 coronary risk factors.

20. A: This patient presents with a classic case of hyperlipidemia with increases in total cholesterol, triglycerides, and LDL-C as well as a low HDL-C. Statins are the drug of first choice in hyperlipidemia due to their efficacy and increased patient compliance. Nicotinic acid is best known for its HDL-elevating effects, although it causes flushing and nausea. Ezetimibe, which is a cholesterol absorption inhibitor, is best used in combination with a statin and is associated with gastrointestinal distress. Niacin and nicotinic acid are the same drug.

21. C: Answer C is true based on several clinical trials. Actually, 50% spontaneously reconvert in 48 hours. The 2,3,4 Cardioversion Rule states if AF fewer than 2 days, cardiovert while on heparin. If AF greater than 2 days, patients must be on oral anticoagulants (OAC) for 3 weeks before

cardioverting. Plus, once the patient has undergone cardioversion, they must continue on OAC for 4 weeks.

22. A: The normal range for TSH is 0.45–4.5 μIU/mL. In primary hypothyroidism, TSH is high while free T3 and free T4 are low. Patients with a TSH of 6-10 μIU/mL have a low risk of developing true hypothyroidism while patients with a TSH greater than 10 μIU/mL are at high risk. Hashimoto's thyroiditis requires the presence of autoimmune antibodies (antiperoxidase, antithyroglobulin).

23. D: Signs of Cushing syndrome consist of central obesity, "moon" facies, hirsutism, menstrual disorders, and glucose intolerance due to an overproduction of cortisol. Graves disease is a form of hyperthyroidism while Addison's disease is due to underproduction of cortisol. Hyperparathyroidism affects the body's regulation of calcium.

24. B: Metformin, a biguanide, is a category B in pregnancy so it is safe to use. Since metformin may cause vitamin B_{12} malabsorption, regular B_{12} monitoring is still necessary. Metformin is safe in older children, but not during breastfeeding.

25. D: Parkinson's is a hypokinetic disorder and marked by 4-6 Hz resting tremors which is the presenting symptom in 50-70% of patients. Postural instability is a late symptom which increases the risk of falls. Dyskinesia and myoclonus are hyperkinetic disorders so are not associated with Parkinson's.

26. A: Complex partial seizures are marked by both altered consciousness and behavior and typically last 1-2 minutes. However, simple partial seizures involve preserved consciousness and the Jacksonian march.

27. D: Antivirals work best when started within 24 to 48 hours of the first sign of influenza symptoms. However, there are still some benefits if started after 48 hours. Amantadine and rimantadine are older antivirals that are not effective against influenza due to increased resistance. Answers A and C are true.

28. B: Acute bronchitis is mostly due to viruses and therefore not responsive to antibiotics. Antibiotics are used in patients listed in C, in acute exacerbations of chronic bronchitis, or if serious complications are suspected due to comorbid conditions. Treatment should focus on supportive care. Studies indicate that bronchodilators may be useful in providing symptom relief for patients with acute bronchitis with wheezing or airflow obstruction.

29. C: Pneumonia is the 6th leading cause of death in the United States. Diagnosis is based on a positive chest x-ray, tachypnea, crackles or rales, fever, and cough. Crackles and rales are only heard in 75-80% of patients with pneumonia and should not be the sole criterion for diagnosis. CURB-65 is a pneumonia severity score based on a 5-point system and can aid the physician in determining inpatient verses outpatient treatment as well as mortality. Scores of 0-1 indicate a low risk and may be treated on an outpatient basis and scores of 2-5 indicate increasing severity and should be admitted to the hospital for treatment. Each of the following is worth 1 point: confusion, BUN greater than 19 mg/dL, RR greater than 30/min, systolic BP less than 90 or diastolic less than 60 mmHg, and age greater than 65 years. With these criteria, the above patient had a score of 1 and C is true. Pneumonia may be treated with either monotherapy or combination therapy and is aimed at treating the pathogen.

30. D: Answer A describes step 2 asthma or mild persistent. Answer B describes step 4 asthma or severe persistent. Answer C describes step 1 asthma or mild intermittent. Answer D is correct and describes step 3 asthma or moderate persistent.

31. C: Answer A is the treatment of choice for step 2 asthma (mild, persistent). Answer B is true for step 1 asthma (intermittent). In step 3 asthma, 2 medications are needed included in those listed in answer C. Finally, answer D refers to the treatment necessary in step 4 asthma (severe persistent). Treatment should be reevaluated every 1 to 6 months.

32. D: All of the above are true for COPD. COPD is the 4th leading cause of death in the United States and is defined as a chronic productive cough that lasts for at least 3 months for 2 consecutive years.

33. B: Testicular torsion is a true emergency and requires swift diagnosis since testicular function decreases with time. The definitive treatment for testicular torsion is surgical detorsion. The pain in testicular torsion typically occurs within hours instead of days as in epididymitis or orchitis. Spermatoceles are typically asymptomatic and develop over time.

34. B: A pelvic examination with a cervical smear and culture should be performed in both primary and secondary dysmenorrhea. B is true. Laparoscopy should be considered in patients who may have endometriosis or underlying pathology, but is not the gold standard for diagnosing dysmenorrhea. Secondary dysmenorrhea typically does not respond well to OCs or NSAIDs, so answer D is false.

35. C: According to medical research, women with abnormal uterine bleeding should receive an endometrial biopsy when they: are over 35 years old, are obese, have prolonged unopposed estrogen stimulation, and have chronic anovulation.

36. C: When diagnosing a woman with abdominal pain, one should rule out gynecologic causes. These causes can be divided into acute and chronic causes in the non-pregnant patient or acute causes in the pregnant patient. Answers A, B, and D are all acute causes, leaving answer C as a chronic cause. Other chronic causes in the non-pregnant patient include dysmenorrhea, Mittelschmerz, and cancer.

37. B: Tricyclic antidepressants, like amitriptyline in answer B, are known for their cardiotoxic side effects, especially in the elderly. SSRIs (selective serotonin reuptake inhibitors), like fluoxetine in answer A, are generally the first-line of therapy due to their safety profile. Also, dopamine reuptake inhibitors and SNRIs (serotonin and norepinephrine reuptake inhibitors), like bupropion and venlafaxine, respectively, are generally safe in the elderly.

38. A: General anxiety disorders (GAD) involve excessive anxiety and worry for at least 6 months and unpredictable events may play a role in developing GAD. Panic disorders involve a sudden onset of fear or discomfort that typically peak within 10 minutes. Social phobias involve anxiety revolving around social or performance situations to the point that they are avoided if at all possible. Specific, or simple, phobias involve irrational anxiety to specific situations or objects like snakes, other animals, flying, or needles. Answer A best describes the patient in this question.

39. D: Somatoform disorders involve unexplained physical symptoms that cannot be linked to underlying medical conditions and cause the patient much distress. Multiple systems are involved, including 4 sites that produce pain, and these symptoms are not willfully produced by the patient. However, malingering is willful and deceptive and typically involves multiple presentations of the same, vague problem. Therefore, answer D is correct.

40. C: Fluoride is important for the primary prevention of dental caries. Fluoride is not required if their primary source for their water supply is greater than 0.6 ppm fluoride ion. Since their fluoride content falls between 0.3-0.6 ppm, fluoride supplements should be 0.25 mg PO qD from 3-6 years old and 0.5 mg PO qD from 6-16 years old. Thus, the answer is C. If water contains less than 0.3

ppm, fluoride supplements should be started at 0.25 mg PO qD between 6 months to 6 years, 0.5 mg PO qD from 3-6 years old, and 1 mg PO qD from 6-16 years old.

41. C: The AAP (American Academy of Pediatrics) released guidelines for the treatment of AOM in February 2013. Patients at least 6 months old with severe signs or symptoms of unilateral or bilateral AOM, like the patient above, should be treated with antibiotics. Also treat patients with antibiotics if they are 6-23 months old with nonsevere, bilateral AOM. High-dose amoxicillin is the first line of treatment in patients without penicillin allergies, without purulent conjunctivitis, and without antibiotic use within the last 30 days. One should only take the wait-and-see approach to patients with nonsevere unilateral AOM if over 23 months old. Therefore, answer C is correct.

42. D: Travelers' diarrhea is usually self-limiting in 3-4 days, so answer A is incorrect. Due to increasing resistance, trimethoprim-sulfamethoxazole and doxycycline are no longer typically recommended, so answer B is incorrect. Also, answer C is incorrect because azithromycin is the drug of choice in resistant Campylobacter infections. Answer D is correct.

43. C: All are true except answer C. Typically patients do not seek help and the hearing loss is only discovered after a loved one or caretaker brings it to the attention of the doctor. The Weber test remains normal as long as long as the hearing loss is symmetric and the Rinne test, which tests for conductive hearing loss, remains normal.

44. A: All of the above, except answer A, are risk factors for developing cataracts. Other risk factors include advancing age, female gender, diabetes, and chronic steroid use. Cataracts involve an opacification and thickening of the lens. It is the leading cause of blindness worldwide.

45. A: These are the first multi-disciplinary, evidence-based practice guidelines of its kind. Tympanostomy tubes are recommended in children as in answer A and in children with unilateral or bilateral OME with associated symptoms like vestibular, behavioral, ear discomfort, or lowered quality of life. Once tympanostomy tubes are placed, patients who develop OM should be treated with only topical antibiotics, so answer C is false. Also, answer D is false because children with tympanostomy tubes may swim or bathe without earplugs.

46. D: All of the above are true except for answer D. In the case of abdominal aneurism screening, an abdominal ultrasound should only be performed once in men who have a history of smoking.

47. E: All of the above are legal factors when one is faced with the diagnosis of or susceptibility to a genetic disorder. Laws are in place to protect the patient's privacy and possible discrimination based on the information found during genetic testing including HIPAA (Health Insurance Portability and Accountability Act) and GINA (Genetic Information Nondiscriminatory Act of 2008). Care needs to be taken to understand these legal issues in the primary care setting.

48. B: Therapeutic alliance refers to the bond that develops between the physician and patient due to the physician's good communication skills as he or she cares for the patient. Medical knowledge alone may not be relied upon to care for the patient so answer B is false. It relies on the physician's ability to impart medical knowledge during the visit so the patient can understand. A good therapeutic alliance helps increase patient adherence, patient satisfaction, and health.

49. E: All of the above are true and the understanding of each is important in establishing culturally competent health care. Other areas to consider include what culturally influenced treatment options the patient seeks and how body signs and symptoms are interpreted.

50. B: All of the above are true except for answer B. The most commonly used opioid in palliative care is morphine, which has many different formulations readily available. Parenteral and oral forms of morphine sulfate supply different doses morphine so one should be careful when converting from one to the other.

Special Report: Basic Review of Types of Fractures

A fracture is defined as a break in a bone that may sometimes involve cartilaginous structures. A fracture can be classified according to its cause or the type of break. The following definitions are used to describe breaks.

1. Traumatic fracture – break in a bone resulting from injury
2. Spontaneous fracture – break in a bone resulting from disease
3. Pathologic fracture – another name for a spontaneous fracture
4. Compound fracture – occurs when fracture bone is exposed to the outside by an opening in the skin
5. Simple fracture - occurs when a break is contained within the skin
6. Greenstick fracture - a traumatic break that is incomplete and occurs on the convex surface of the bend in the bone
7. Fissured fracture – a traumatic break that involves an incomplete longitudinal break
8. Comminuted fracture – a traumatic break that involves a complete fracture that results in several bony fragments
9. Transverse fracture – a traumatic break that is complete and occurs at a right angle to the axis of the bone
10. Oblique fracture- a traumatic break that occurs at an angle other than a right angel to the axis of the bone.
11. Spiral fracture – a traumatic break that occurs by twisting a bone with extreme force

A compound fracture is much more dangerous than a simple break. This is due to the break in skin that can allow microorganisms to infect the injured tissue. When a fracture occurs, blood vessels within the bone and its periosteum are disrupted. The periosteum, covering of fibrous connective tissue on the surface of the bone, may also be damaged or torn.

Special Report: Quick Reference Lesion Review

Occipital Lobe	Homonymous hemianopsia, partial seizures with limited visual phenomena
Thalamus	Contralateral thalamus pain, contralateral hemisensory loss
Pineal gland	Early hydrocephalus, papillary abnormalities, Parinaud's syndrome
Internal capsule	Hemisensory loss, homonymous hemianopsia, contralateral hemiplegia
Basal ganglia	Contralateral dystonia, Contralateral choreoathetosis
Pons	Diplopia, internal strabismus, VI and VII involvement, contralateral hemisensory and hemiparesis loss, issilateral cerebellar ataxia
Broca's area	Motor dysphasia
Precentral gyrus	Jacksonian seizures, generalized seizures, hemiparesis
Superficial parietal lobe	Receptive dysphasia
Cerebellar hemisphere	Ipsilateral cerebellar ataxia with hypotonia, dysmetria, intention tremor, nystagmus to side of lesion
Midbrain	Loss of upward gaze, III involvement, ipsilateral cerebellar signs, diplopia
Angular gyrus	Finger agnosia, allochiria, agraphia, acalculia
Temporal lobe	Contralateral homonymous upper quadrantanopsia, partial complex seizures
Paracentral lobe	Urgency of micturition, incontinence, progressive spastic paraparesis
Third Ventricle	Hydrocephalus
Fourth Ventricle	Hydrocephalus, progressive spastic hemiparesis
Optic Chiasm	Bitemporal hemianopsia, optic atrophy
Uncus	Partial complex seizures
Superior temporal gyrus	Receptive dysphasia
Prefrontal area	Apathy, poor attention span, loss of judgement, release phenomena, distractible
Orbital surface frontal lobe	Paroxysmal atrial tachycardia
Hypothalmus	Amenorrhea, cachexia, hypopituitarism, hypothyrodism, impotence, diencephalic autonomic seizures

Special Report: High Frequency Terms

The following terms were compiled as high frequency terms. I recommend printing out this list and identifying the terms you are unfamiliar with. Then, use a medical dictionary or the internet to look up the terms you have questions about. Take one section per day if you have the time to maximize recall.

A

Acquired immunodeficiency syndrome
Acromegaly
Acute lymphoblastic leukemia
Acute myelogenous leukemia
Acute nonlymphocytic leukemia
Adenocarcinoma
Adjuvant disease
Agoraphobia
Alopecia
Alzheimer's dementia
Amebiasis
Amenorrhea
Amyloidosis
Anastomoses
Aneurysm
Angina pectoris
Angiogenesis
Anklyosing spondylitis
Anxiety
Appendicitis
Arterial disease
Arteriosclerosis
Arthralgia
Arthritis bacterial
Arthritis (Crohn's disease)
Arthritis (gouty)
Arthritis (Reiter's syndrome)
Arthritis (Rheumatoid arthritis
Atypical angina
Avascular necrosis
AZT

B

Barrett's oesophagus
Back pain (Sciatica)
Back pain (tumor)
Barlow's syndrome
Basal cell carcinoma
Behçet's disease
Benign prostate hypertrophy
Biliary disease
Bilirubin
Biliverdin
Blood cultures
Boerhaave's syndrome
Bornholm disease
Bowen's disease
Bradycardia
Braxton-Hicks contractions
Bronchiectasis
Budd-Chiari syndrome
Buerger's disease
Bulimia
Burkitt Lymphoma

C

CAD
Cancer (basal cell)
Cancer (pancreatic)
Cancer (prostate)
Cancer (squamous cell)
Candidiasis
Cardiac disease
Cardiac valvular disease
Carpal tunnel syndrome
Catecholamines
Cauda equina syndrome
Centriacinar emphysema
Charcot-Marie-Tooth disease
Chest pain
Chest x-ray
Cholecystectomy
Cholecystitis
Chondroma
Chronic lymphocytic leukemia
Chronic myelogenous leukemia
Chvostek's sign
Cirrhosis
Click-murmur syndrome
Clonidine
Coccygodynia
COLD

Colles' fracture
Combined hormone replacement
Computed tomography (CT) scan of head
Confusion
Conjunctivitis
Connective tissue disease
Conn's syndrome
Coombs' test
Cor pulmonale
Corticosteroids
CREST syndrome
Cretinism
Creutzfeldt-Jakob disease
Crohn's disease
Cushing's syndrome

D

Dactylitis
Degenerative heart disease
Dermatitis
Diabetes insipidus
Diabetes mellitus
Diabetic nephropathy
Dialysis
Diaphoresis
Dietary modification
Diffuse lymphoma
Digitalis
Dopamine
Down's syndrome
Duchenne muscular dystrophy
DVT
Dysmenorrhea
Dyspnea

E

Ecchymosis
Ectopic pregnancy
Electrocardiogram (ECG)
Embolism
Emphysema
Encephalopathy
Endocrine system
Epinephrine
Epstein-Barr virus
Erythropoietien
Erythema nodosum
Esophagitis
Ewing's sarcoma
Exophthalmos

F

Fabry's disease
Fallopian tube
Fallot's tetralogy
Fanconi's syndrome
Fatigue
Fecal incontinence
Fibrillation
Fibromyalgia syndrome
Fibrous ankylosis
Follicle-stimulating hormone
Fuch's corneal dystrophy
Full blood count (FBC)
Functional dyspepsia

G

Gamma globulin
Gangrene
Gaucher's disease
Gestatoin
Giant cell tumor
Gilbert's syndrome
Gliosis
Glucagon
Glucose tolerance test
Goodpasture's syndrome
Graves disease
Guillai-Barre' syndrome
Gynecomastia

H

Haemochromatosis
Hand-foot syndrome
Hashimoto's thyroiditis
Hartmann's solution
Heart failure
Heart rate
Helper T cells
Hemarthrosis
Hematuria
Hemophilia
Hemorrhage
Henoch-Schönlein syndrome
Heparin
Hepatic encephalopathy
Hepatitis (A-E)

Herpes zoster
Hiatal hernia
Hirschsprung's disease
HIV
Hodgkin's disease
Homans sign
Homocystinuria
Hormone replacement therapy
Huntington's chorea
Hurler's syndrome
Hunter's syndrome
Hyalinization
Hypercortisolism
Hyperglycemia
Hyperplasia
Hyperparathyroidism
Hypnotic preparations
Hypochromia
Hyponatremia
Hypothyroidism
Hypoxia
Hysterectomy

I

IBD Inflammatory bowel disease
IBS Irritable bowel syndrome
Immune serum globulin
Immunoglobulins (IgE, IgG, IgM)
Inderal
Induration
Infectious arthritis
Inflammatory bowel disease
Inhibitors
Interferon
Interleukin (I), (II)
Interstitial cystitis
Intramedullary tumors
Iridocyclitis
Ischemic Heart Disease
Isographs
Isotonic solution

J

Jaundice
Joint pain (gout)
Joint pain (psoriatic arthritis)
Joint sepsis
Jevenile rheumatoid arthritis

K

Kaposi's sarcoma
Kawasaki disease
Kehr's sign
Kernicterus
Ketoacidosis
Kidney failure
Kidney stones
Kleihauer test
Korsakoff's psychosis
Krabbe's disease
Kreim test
Kupffer's cells
Kussmaul's respirations

L

Labile hypertension
Lactation
Large cell carcinoma
Lesch-Nyhan syndrome
Leukemias
Leukopenia
Lewy body dementia
Lhermitte's sign
Lipoproteins
Lobar pneumonia
Low back pain
Low density lipoprotein
Lumbar pain
Lupus carditis
Lupus erythematosus
Lyme disease
Lymph nodes
Lymphocyctes
Lymphoid cells
Lymphotoxin

M

Macrophages
Malignant melanoma
Mallory-Weiss tear
Mantoux test
Marie-Strumpell disease
Mastodynia
Meckel's diverticulum
Medial cartilage tear
Melanoma
Menarche

N

O

P

Q

R

S

T

U

V

W

CPR Guidelines for Professional Rescuers

Topic	Adult	Child	Infant
	Past puberty	1 y/o - puberty	Under 1 y/o
Conscious Choking	abdominal thrusts (or chest thrusts in pregnant/obese)	abdominal thrusts	5 back slaps and 5 chest thrusts in infant
Unconscious Choking	Begin chest compression. Look in the victim's mouth for foreign body before giving breaths.		
Rescue Breaths Normal breath given over 1 second until chest rises.	10-12 breaths per minute (1 breath every 6-8 seconds)	12-20 breaths per minute (1 breath every 3-5 seconds)	20 breaths per minute (1 breath every 3 seconds)
Chest Compressions to Ventilation Ratios (Single Rescuer)	30:2		
Chest Compressions to Ventilation Ratios (Two Rescuer)	30:2	15:2	
Chest Compression rate	At least 100/minute		
Chest Compression Land Marking Method	two hands center of the chest, even with nipples	one hand center of the chest even with nipples	2 or 3 fingers, just below the nipple line at the center of the chest
Chest Compression Depth	At least 2" compression (hands overlapping)	about 2" compression or 1/3 the AP diameter (only heel of one hand)	about 1 ½" compression or 1/3 the AP diameter (2 fingers)
Activate Emergency Response System	As soon as you realize that the victim is unresponsive	After 5 cycles of CPR	After 5 cycles of CPR

Checklist:

- Check the scene
- Check for responsiveness – ask, "Are you OK?"
- Adult - call 911, then administer CPR
- Child/Infant – administer CPR for 5 cycles, then call 911
- Open victim's airway and check for breathing
- Two rescue breaths should be given, 1 second each, and should produce a visible chest rise
- If the air does not go in, reposition and try 2 breaths again
- Check victim's pulse – chest compressions are recommended if an infant or child has a rate less than 60 per minute with signs of poor perfusion
- Continue 30:2 ratio until victim moves, AED is brought to the scene, or professional help arrives

How to Overcome Test Anxiety

Just the thought of taking a test is enough to make most people a little nervous. A test is an important event that can have a long-term impact on your future, so it's important to take it seriously and it's natural to feel anxious about performing well. But just because anxiety is normal, that doesn't mean that it's helpful in test taking, or that you should simply accept it as part of your life. Anxiety can have a variety of effects. These effects can be mild, like making you feel slightly nervous, or severe, like blocking your ability to focus or remember even a simple detail.

If you experience test anxiety—whether severe or mild—it's important to know how to beat it. To discover this, first you need to understand what causes test anxiety.

Causes of Test Anxiety

While we often think of anxiety as an uncontrollable emotional state, it can actually be caused by simple, practical things. One of the most common causes of test anxiety is that a person does not feel adequately prepared for their test. This feeling can be the result of many different issues such as poor study habits or lack of organization, but the most common culprit is time management. Starting to study too late, failing to organize your study time to cover all of the material, or being distracted while you study will mean that you're not well prepared for the test. This may lead to cramming the night before, which will cause you to be physically and mentally exhausted for the test. Poor time management also contributes to feelings of stress, fear, and hopelessness as you realize you are not well prepared but don't know what to do about it.

Other times, test anxiety is not related to your preparation for the test but comes from unresolved fear. This may be a past failure on a test, or poor performance on tests in general. It may come from comparing yourself to others who seem to be performing better or from the stress of living up to expectations. Anxiety may be driven by fears of the future—how failure on this test would affect your educational and career goals. These fears are often completely irrational, but they can still negatively impact your test performance.

Review Video: 3 Reasons You Have Test Anxiety
Visit mometrix.com/academy and enter code: 428468

Elements of Test Anxiety

As mentioned earlier, test anxiety is considered to be an emotional state, but it has physical and mental components as well. Sometimes you may not even realize that you are suffering from test anxiety until you notice the physical symptoms. These can include trembling hands, rapid heartbeat, sweating, nausea, and tense muscles. Extreme anxiety may lead to fainting or vomiting. Obviously, any of these symptoms can have a negative impact on testing. It is important to recognize them as soon as they begin to occur so that you can address the problem before it damages your performance.

Review Video: 3 Ways to Tell You Have Test Anxiety
Visit mometrix.com/academy and enter code: 927847

The mental components of test anxiety include trouble focusing and inability to remember learned information. During a test, your mind is on high alert, which can help you recall information and stay focused for an extended period of time. However, anxiety interferes with your mind's natural processes, causing you to blank out, even on the questions you know well. The strain of testing during anxiety makes it difficult to stay focused, especially on a test that may take several hours. Extreme anxiety can take a huge mental toll, making it difficult not only to recall test information but even to understand the test questions or pull your thoughts together.

Review Video: How Test Anxiety Affects Memory
Visit mometrix.com/academy and enter code: 609003

Effects of Test Anxiety

Test anxiety is like a disease—if left untreated, it will get progressively worse. Anxiety leads to poor performance, and this reinforces the feelings of fear and failure, which in turn lead to poor performances on subsequent tests. It can grow from a mild nervousness to a crippling condition. If allowed to progress, test anxiety can have a big impact on your schooling, and consequently on your future.

Test anxiety can spread to other parts of your life. Anxiety on tests can become anxiety in any stressful situation, and blanking on a test can turn into panicking in a job situation. But fortunately, you don't have to let anxiety rule your testing and determine your grades. There are a number of relatively simple steps you can take to move past anxiety and function normally on a test and in the rest of life.

Review Video: How Test Anxiety Impacts Your Grades
Visit mometrix.com/academy and enter code: 939819

Physical Steps for Beating Test Anxiety

While test anxiety is a serious problem, the good news is that it can be overcome. It doesn't have to control your ability to think and remember information. While it may take time, you can begin taking steps today to beat anxiety.

Just as your first hint that you may be struggling with anxiety comes from the physical symptoms, the first step to treating it is also physical. Rest is crucial for having a clear, strong mind. If you are tired, it is much easier to give in to anxiety. But if you establish good sleep habits, your body and mind will be ready to perform optimally, without the strain of exhaustion. Additionally, sleeping well helps you to retain information better, so you're more likely to recall the answers when you see the test questions.

Getting good sleep means more than going to bed on time. It's important to allow your brain time to relax. Take study breaks from time to time so it doesn't get overworked, and don't study right before bed. Take time to rest your mind before trying to rest your body, or you may find it difficult to fall asleep.

Review Video: The Importance of Sleep for Your Brain
Visit mometrix.com/academy and enter code: 319338

Along with sleep, other aspects of physical health are important in preparing for a test. Good nutrition is vital for good brain function. Sugary foods and drinks may give a burst of energy but this burst is followed by a crash, both physically and emotionally. Instead, fuel your body with protein and vitamin-rich foods.

Also, drink plenty of water. Dehydration can lead to headaches and exhaustion, especially if your brain is already under stress from the rigors of the test. Particularly if your test is a long one, drink water during the breaks. And if possible, take an energy-boosting snack to eat between sections.

Review Video: How Diet Can Affect your Mood
Visit mometrix.com/academy and enter code: 624317

Along with sleep and diet, a third important part of physical health is exercise. Maintaining a steady workout schedule is helpful, but even taking 5-minute study breaks to walk can help get your blood pumping faster and clear your head. Exercise also releases endorphins, which contribute to a positive feeling and can help combat test anxiety.

When you nurture your physical health, you are also contributing to your mental health. If your body is healthy, your mind is much more likely to be healthy as well. So take time to rest, nourish your body with healthy food and water, and get moving as much as possible. Taking these physical steps will make you stronger and more able to take the mental steps necessary to overcome test anxiety.

Review Video: How to Stay Healthy and Prevent Test Anxiety
Visit mometrix.com/academy and enter code: 877894

Mental Steps for Beating Test Anxiety

Working on the mental side of test anxiety can be more challenging, but as with the physical side, there are clear steps you can take to overcome it. As mentioned earlier, test anxiety often stems from lack of preparation, so the obvious solution is to prepare for the test. Effective studying may be the most important weapon you have for beating test anxiety, but you can and should employ several other mental tools to combat fear.

First, boost your confidence by reminding yourself of past success—tests or projects that you aced. If you're putting as much effort into preparing for this test as you did for those, there's no reason you should expect to fail here. Work hard to prepare; then trust your preparation.

Second, surround yourself with encouraging people. It can be helpful to find a study group, but be sure that the people you're around will encourage a positive attitude. If you spend time with others who are anxious or cynical, this will only contribute to your own anxiety. Look for others who are motivated to study hard from a desire to succeed, not from a fear of failure.

Third, reward yourself. A test is physically and mentally tiring, even without anxiety, and it can be helpful to have something to look forward to. Plan an activity following the test, regardless of the outcome, such as going to a movie or getting ice cream.

When you are taking the test, if you find yourself beginning to feel anxious, remind yourself that you know the material. Visualize successfully completing the test. Then take a few deep, relaxing breaths and return to it. Work through the questions carefully but with confidence, knowing that you are capable of succeeding.

Developing a healthy mental approach to test taking will also aid in other areas of life. Test anxiety affects more than just the actual test—it can be damaging to your mental health and even contribute to depression. It's important to beat test anxiety before it becomes a problem for more than testing.

Review Video: Test Anxiety and Depression
Visit mometrix.com/academy and enter code: 904704

Study Strategy

Being prepared for the test is necessary to combat anxiety, but what does being prepared look like? You may study for hours on end and still not feel prepared. What you need is a strategy for test prep. The next few pages outline our recommended steps to help you plan out and conquer the challenge of preparation.

Step 1: Scope Out the Test

Learn everything you can about the format (multiple choice, essay, etc.) and what will be on the test. Gather any study materials, course outlines, or sample exams that may be available. Not only will this help you to prepare, but knowing what to expect can help to alleviate test anxiety.

Step 2: Map Out the Material

Look through the textbook or study guide and make note of how many chapters or sections it has. Then divide these over the time you have. For example, if a book has 15 chapters and you have five days to study, you need to cover three chapters each day. Even better, if you have the time, leave an extra day at the end for overall review after you have gone through the material in depth.

If time is limited, you may need to prioritize the material. Look through it and make note of which sections you think you already have a good grasp on, and which need review. While you are studying, skim quickly through the familiar sections and take more time on the challenging parts. Write out your plan so you don't get lost as you go. Having a written plan also helps you feel more in control of the study, so anxiety is less likely to arise from feeling overwhelmed at the amount to cover. A sample plan may look like this:

- Day 1: Skim chapters 1–4, study chapter 5 (especially pages 31–33)
- Day 2: Study chapters 6–7, skim chapters 8–9
- Day 3: Skim chapter 10, study chapters 11–12 (especially pages 87–90)
- Day 4: Study chapters 13–15
- Day 5: Overall review (focus most on chapters 5, 6, and 12), take practice test

Step 3: Gather Your Tools

Decide what study method works best for you. Do you prefer to highlight in the book as you study and then go back over the highlighted portions? Or do you type out notes of the important information? Or is it helpful to make flashcards that you can carry with you? Assemble the pens, index cards, highlighters, post-it notes, and any other materials you may need so you won't be distracted by getting up to find things while you study.

If you're having a hard time retaining the information or organizing your notes, experiment with different methods. For example, try color-coding by subject with colored pens, highlighters, or post-it notes. If you learn better by hearing, try recording yourself reading your notes so you can listen while in the car, working out, or simply sitting at your desk. Ask a friend to quiz you from your flashcards, or try teaching someone the material to solidify it in your mind.

Step 4: Create Your Environment

It's important to avoid distractions while you study. This includes both the obvious distractions like visitors and the subtle distractions like an uncomfortable chair (or a too-comfortable couch that makes you want to fall asleep). Set up the best study environment possible: good lighting and a comfortable work area. If background music helps you focus, you may want to turn it on, but otherwise keep the room quiet. If you are using a computer to take notes, be sure you don't have any other windows open, especially applications like social media, games, or anything else that could distract you. Silence your phone and turn off notifications. Be sure to keep water close by so you stay hydrated while you study (but avoid unhealthy drinks and snacks).

Also, take into account the best time of day to study. Are you freshest first thing in the morning? Try to set aside some time then to work through the material. Is your mind clearer in the afternoon or evening? Schedule your study session then. Another method is to study at the same time of day that you will take the test, so that your brain gets used to working on the material at that time and will be ready to focus at test time.

Step 5: Study!

Once you have done all the study preparation, it's time to settle into the actual studying. Sit down, take a few moments to settle your mind so you can focus, and begin to follow your study plan. Don't give in to distractions or let yourself procrastinate. This is your time to prepare so you'll be ready to fearlessly approach the test. Make the most of the time and stay focused.

Of course, you don't want to burn out. If you study too long you may find that you're not retaining the information very well. Take regular study breaks. For example, taking five minutes out of every hour to walk briskly, breathing deeply and swinging your arms, can help your mind stay fresh.

As you get to the end of each chapter or section, it's a good idea to do a quick review. Remind yourself of what you learned and work on any difficult parts. When you feel that you've mastered the material, move on to the next part. At the end of your study session, briefly skim through your notes again.

But while review is helpful, cramming last minute is NOT. If at all possible, work ahead so that you won't need to fit all your study into the last day. Cramming overloads your brain with more information than it can process and retain, and your tired mind may struggle to recall even previously learned information when it is overwhelmed with last-minute study. Also, the urgent nature of cramming and the stress placed on your brain contribute to anxiety. You'll be more likely to go to the test feeling unprepared and having trouble thinking clearly.

So don't cram, and don't stay up late before the test, even just to review your notes at a leisurely pace. Your brain needs rest more than it needs to go over the information again. In fact, plan to finish your studies by noon or early afternoon the day before the test. Give your brain the rest of the day to relax or focus on other things, and get a good night's sleep. Then you will be fresh for the test and better able to recall what you've studied.

Step 6: Take a practice test

Many courses offer sample tests, either online or in the study materials. This is an excellent resource to check whether you have mastered the material, as well as to prepare for the test format and environment.

Check the test format ahead of time: the number of questions, the type (multiple choice, free response, etc.), and the time limit. Then create a plan for working through them. For example, if you have 30 minutes to take a 60-question test, your limit is 30 seconds per question. Spend less time on the questions you know well so that you can take more time on the difficult ones.

If you have time to take several practice tests, take the first one open book, with no time limit. Work through the questions at your own pace and make sure you fully understand them. Gradually work up to taking a test under test conditions: sit at a desk with all study materials put away and set a timer. Pace yourself to make sure you finish the test with time to spare and go back to check your answers if you have time.

After each test, check your answers. On the questions you missed, be sure you understand why you missed them. Did you misread the question (tests can use tricky wording)? Did you forget the information? Or was it something you hadn't learned? Go back and study any shaky areas that the practice tests reveal.

Taking these tests not only helps with your grade, but also aids in combating test anxiety. If you're already used to the test conditions, you're less likely to worry about it, and working through tests until you're scoring well gives you a confidence boost. Go through the practice tests until you feel comfortable, and then you can go into the test knowing that you're ready for it.

Test Tips

On test day, you should be confident, knowing that you've prepared well and are ready to answer the questions. But aside from preparation, there are several test day strategies you can employ to maximize your performance.

First, as stated before, get a good night's sleep the night before the test (and for several nights before that, if possible). Go into the test with a fresh, alert mind rather than staying up late to study.

Try not to change too much about your normal routine on the day of the test. It's important to eat a nutritious breakfast, but if you normally don't eat breakfast at all, consider eating just a protein bar. If you're a coffee drinker, go ahead and have your normal coffee. Just make sure you time it so that the caffeine doesn't wear off right in the middle of your test. Avoid sugary beverages, and drink enough water to stay hydrated but not so much that you need a restroom break 10 minutes into the test. If your test isn't first thing in the morning, consider going for a walk or doing a light workout before the test to get your blood flowing.

Allow yourself enough time to get ready, and leave for the test with plenty of time to spare so you won't have the anxiety of scrambling to arrive in time. Another reason to be early is to select a good seat. It's helpful to sit away from doors and windows, which can be distracting. Find a good seat, get out your supplies, and settle your mind before the test begins.

When the test begins, start by going over the instructions carefully, even if you already know what to expect. Make sure you avoid any careless mistakes by following the directions.

Then begin working through the questions, pacing yourself as you've practiced. If you're not sure on an answer, don't spend too much time on it, and don't let it shake your confidence. Either skip it and come back later, or eliminate as many wrong answers as possible and guess among the remaining ones. Don't dwell on these questions as you continue—put them out of your mind and focus on what lies ahead.

Be sure to read all of the answer choices, even if you're sure the first one is the right answer. Sometimes you'll find a better one if you keep reading. But don't second-guess yourself if you do immediately know the answer. Your gut instinct is usually right. Don't let test anxiety rob you of the information you know.

If you have time at the end of the test (and if the test format allows), go back and review your answers. Be cautious about changing any, since your first instinct tends to be correct, but make sure you didn't misread any of the questions or accidentally mark the wrong answer choice. Look over any you skipped and make an educated guess.

At the end, leave the test feeling confident. You've done your best, so don't waste time worrying about your performance or wishing you could change anything. Instead, celebrate the successful completion of this test. And finally, use this test to learn how to deal with anxiety even better next time.

Review Video: 5 Tips to Beat Test Anxiety
Visit mometrix.com/academy and enter code: 570656

Important Qualification

Not all anxiety is created equal. If your test anxiety is causing major issues in your life beyond the classroom or testing center, or if you are experiencing troubling physical symptoms related to your anxiety, it may be a sign of a serious physiological or psychological condition. If this sounds like your situation, we strongly encourage you to seek professional help.

Thank You

We at Mometrix would like to extend our heartfelt thanks to you, our friend and patron, for allowing us to play a part in your journey. It is a privilege to serve people from all walks of life who are unified in their commitment to building the best future they can for themselves.

The preparation you devote to these important testing milestones may be the most valuable educational opportunity you have for making a real difference in your life. We encourage you to put your heart into it—that feeling of succeeding, overcoming, and yes, conquering will be well worth the hours you've invested.

We want to hear your story, your struggles and your successes, and if you see any opportunities for us to improve our materials so we can help others even more effectively in the future, please share that with us as well. **The team at Mometrix would be absolutely thrilled to hear from you!** So please, send us an email (support@mometrix.com) and let's stay in touch.

If you'd like some additional help, check out these other resources we offer for your exam:

http://MometrixFlashcards.com/FamilyPractice

Additional Bonus Material

Due to our efforts to try to keep this book to a manageable length, we've created a link that will give you access to all of your additional bonus material.

Please visit **https://www.mometrix.com/bonus948/familypractice** to access the information.